This book is edited and designed by the Editorial Committee of *Cultural China* series

Text by Guo Changqing
Translation by Cao Jianxin
Cover and Interior Design by Wang Wei

Assistant Editor: Cao Yue
Copy Editor: Kirstin Mattson
Editors: Yang Xiaohe, Wu Yuezhou
Editorial Director: Zhang Yicong

Senior Consultants: Sun Yong, Wu Ying, Yang Xinci
Managing Director and Publisher: Wang Youbu

ISBN: 978-1-60220-025-8

Address any comments about *The Complete Guide of Self-Massage: A Natural Way for Prevention and Treatment through Traditional Chinese Medicine* to:

Better Link Press
99 Park Ave
New York, NY 10016
USA

or

Shanghai Press and Publishing Development Company, Ltd.
F 7 Donghu Road, Shanghai, China (200031)
Email: comments_betterlinkpress@hotmail.com

Printed in China by Shenzhen Donnelley Printing Co., Ltd.
1   3   5   7   9   10   8   6   4   2

The Complete Guide of
SELF-MASSAGE
A Natural Way for
Prevention and Treatment through
Traditional Chinese Medicine

By Guo Changqing

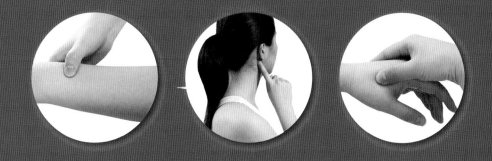

Better Link Press

Contents

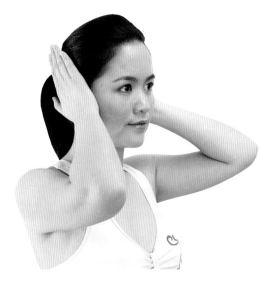

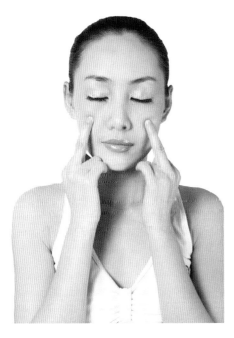

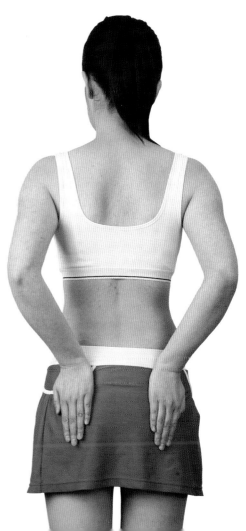

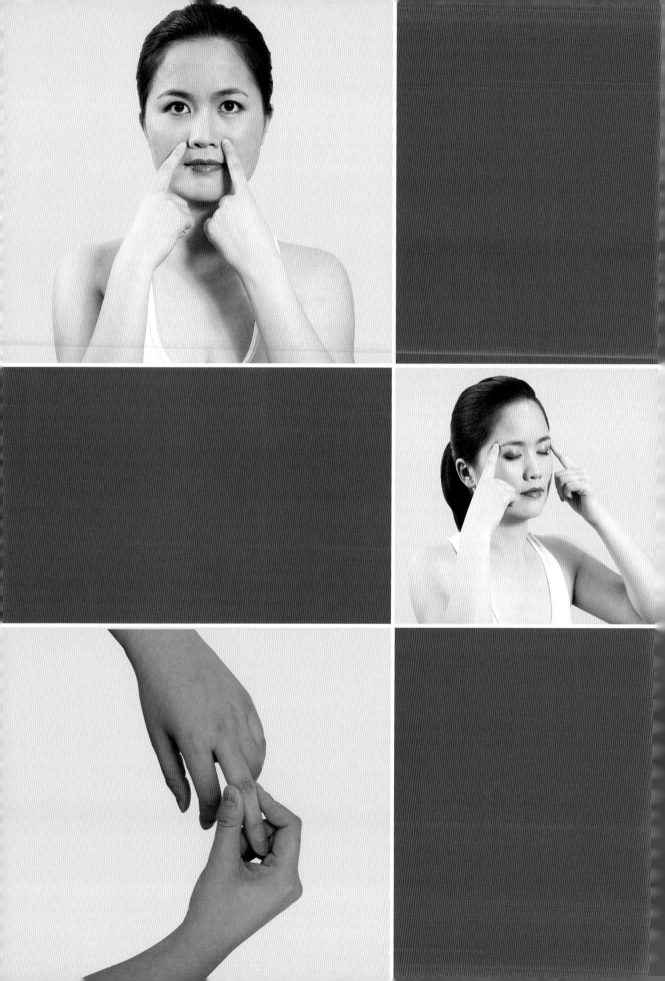

PREFACE

Acupoint massage is truly one of the most vital, effective and multifaceted techniques in traditional Chinese medicine (TCM). It refers to the various ways in which touch is used to stimulate different acupoints, specific locations on the body through which the circulation of qi (vital energy) and blood can be manipulated.

By regulating these life energies we can ease pain, calm the mind, and enhance health and beauty. Through curing and preventing disease, acupoint massage is a key to increased longevity, and a happier and healthier life.

By using the hands, we can exert force on certain acupoints to convey curative effects deep into the body. This occurs due to the routes of meridians and collaterals within the body, which serve as channels for the flow of qi, reaching from external points all the way to the internal organs.

By influencing the correct channels, we can bring qi into affected areas, adjust the balance of yin and yang within the organs, and regulate qi and blood. In this way acupoint massage will cultivate positive energy within the body, dispelling any harmful elements and protecting against disease.

To help you master the TCM therapy of acupoint massage, I have called upon the experience of my predecessors in combination with my clinical practice of many years. Through explanations and descriptions accompanied by many illustrations and diagrams, I have compiled an easy-to-understand reference book describing the recommended acupoint massage to be used for a vast variety of common ailments.

This book first provides some basic information so that you will become familiar with meridians, collaterals and acupoints, as well as some of the underlying theory of TCM related to this therapy. You will learn how to quickly and accurately find acupoints as well as be introduced to various massage techniques.

The main content of this book is related to the treatment of common diseases, ranging from minor problems, such as hiccups or a stiff neck, to major ones including diabetes, kidney disorders and infertility. There are also easy therapies for dealing with issues regarding external appearance that trouble many of us, including acne, wrinkles and dark under-eye circles.

Acupoints are amazing! By kneading, pressing, pinching or otherwise manipulating these small targeted areas of the body, we can create a major influence on health and beauty from the inside out. So let's get started with some wonderful healing massage.

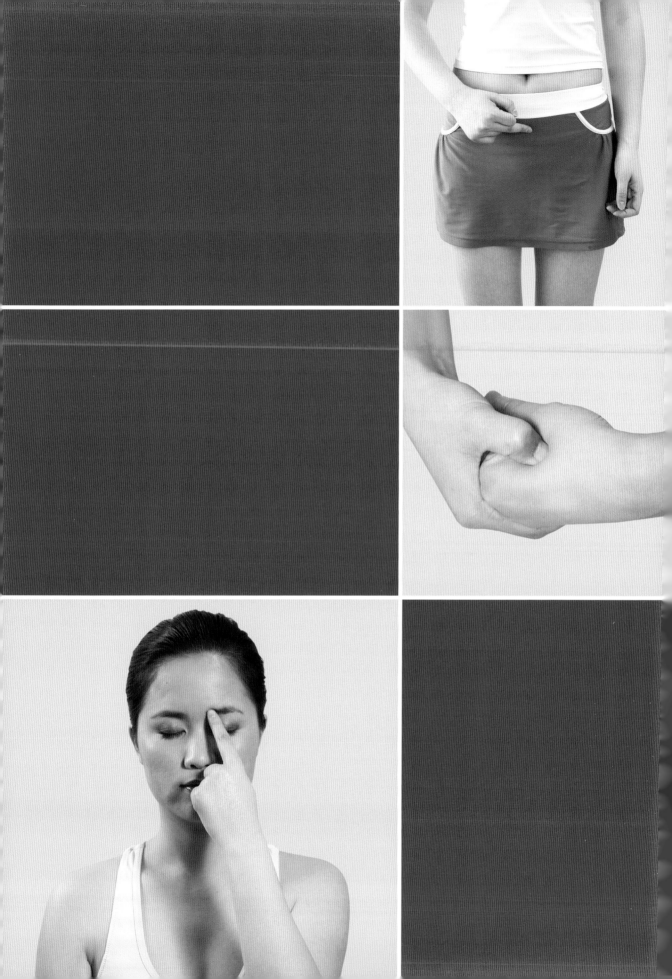

CHAPTER ONE
Introduction to Meridians, Collaterals and Acupoints

In the theoretical system of traditional Chinese medicine, meridians and collaterals are regarded as a system that makes connections throughout the body, working their way from external points to the five internal organs (as defined by TCM) and viscera. The meridians and collaterals that run throughout the whole body serve to transport qi and blood, nourish muscles and bones.

1. Meridians and Collaterals

Meridians are the system's major channels, and they run across the body vertically. Meridians may then branch out into finer channels called collaterals which can connect the meridians throughout the body.

In the human body there are twelve meridians, each with its own two-letter code for easy reference:
- Taiyin Lung Meridian of Hand (LU)
- Jueyin Pericardium Meridian of Hand (PC)
- Shaoyin Heart Meridian of Hand (HT)
- Yangming Large Intestine Meridian of Hand (LI)
- Shaoyang Sanjiao Meridian of Hand (SJ)
- Taiyang Small Intestine Meridian of Hand (SI)
- Yangming Stomach Meridian of Foot (ST)
- Shaoyang Gallbladder Meridian of Foot (GB)
- Taiyang Bladder Meridian of Foot (BL)
- Taiyin Spleen Meridian of Foot (SP)
- Jueyin Liver Meridian of Foot (LV)
- Shaoyin Kidney Meridian of Foot (KI).

In addition there is the Conception Vessel (RN) running vertically in the front of the body and Governing Vessel (DU) at the back.

Naming conventions for meridians and collaterals:
- Those distributed in the upper limbs are called "hand meridians" while those in the lower limbs are called "foot meridians."
- According to TCM the back is associated with yang while the abdomen is concerned with yin, and the outside is concerned with yang while the inside is associated with yin. Therefore yang channels are mostly distributed in the back and the outside of the limbs, while yin channels are mostly distributed in the abdomen and inner side of the limbs. You will see "yin" in the name of the meridians running

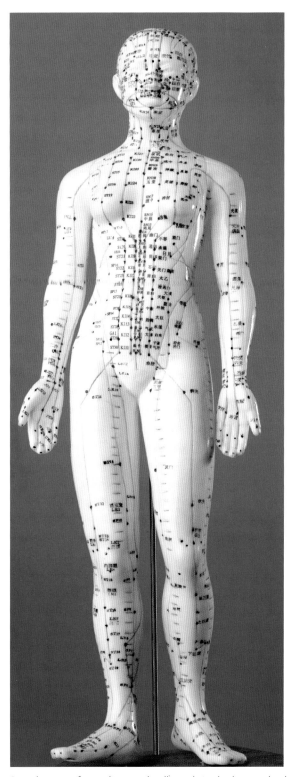

Distribution of meridians and collaterals in the human body.

inside the limb (for example, Taiyin Meridian) while "yang" appears in the name of meridians running on the outside (for example, Taiyang Meridian).

• Meridians and collaterals are named after related internal organs. According to TCM the five main organs are the heart, liver, spleen, lungs and kidneys. The six viscera include the gallbladder, stomach, small intestine, large intestine, urinary bladder and Sanjiao, in addition to the pericardium. The heart meridian and pericardium meridian are both related to the heart, and the Sanjiao, as described in TCM, comprises three compartments in the trunk of the body.

2. Defining Acupoints ("Shu Points")

Closely related to meridians and collaterals, acupoints are mostly distributed along the routes of meridians and collaterals.

In traditional Chinese medicine, acupoints are called "Shu points," meaning that they are points where acupuncture and moxibustion can be applied. Since these points are densely concentrated with nerve endings or quite thick nerve fibers, they will emit signals when one feels discomfort or pain.

To understand Shu points you must not picture isolated points on the surface of the body. Rather they are closely associated with tissues and inner organs deep within. Due to these connections, Shu points are reaction points for diseases and stimulation points for treatment.

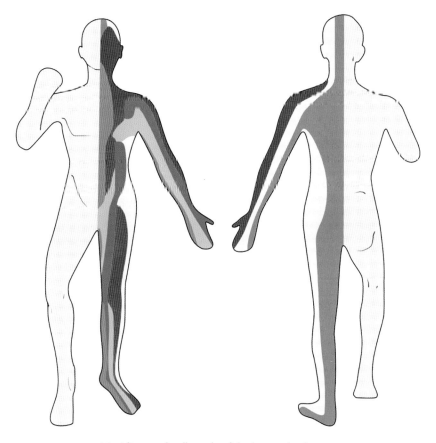

Meridians and collaterals of the human body.

Color of Skin Zone	Sub-Category	Meridian	Treats
	Taiyang	Bladder Meridian of Foot	Kidney system
		Small Intestine Meridian of Hand	Heart system
	Yangming	Large Intestine Meridian of Hand	Lung system
		Stomach Meridian of Foot	Spleen system
	Shaoyang	Gallbladder Meridian of Foot	Liver system
		San Jiao Meridian of Hand	Heart system
	Taiyin	Lung Meridian of Hand	Lung system
		Spleen Meridian of Foot	Spleen system
	Shaoyin	Heart Meridian of Hand	Heart system
		Kidney Meridian of Foot	Kidney system
	Jueyin	Liver Meridian of Foot	Liver system
		Pericardium Meridian of Hand	Heart system

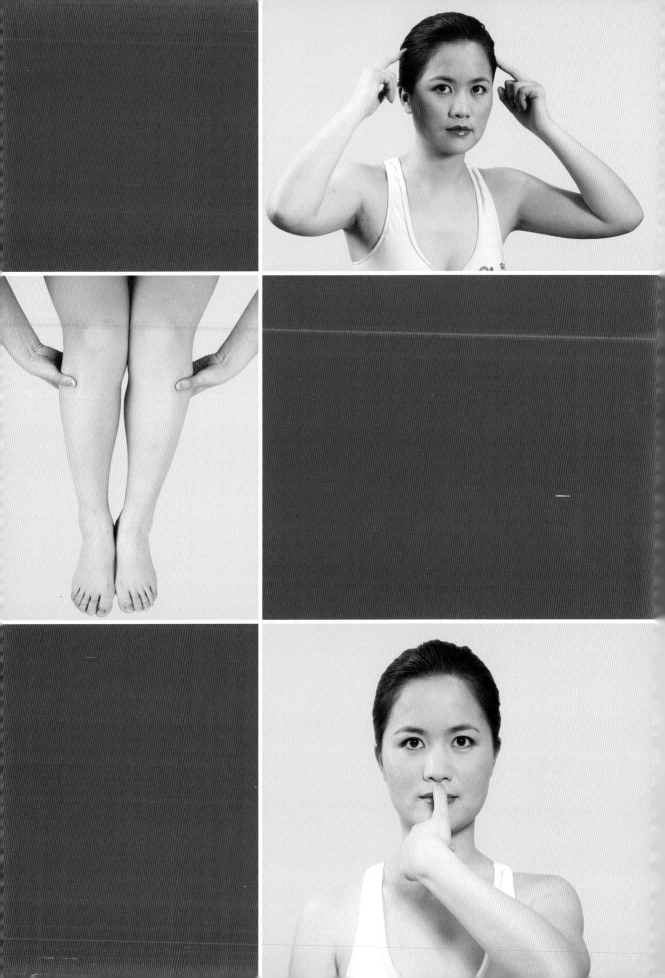

CHAPTER TWO
Acupoint Massage Techniques

Massage serves to directly or indirectly stimulate muscles, bones, joints, ligaments, nerves and blood vessels to produce either a specific or systemic reaction. This functions through the conduction of acupoints, meridians, collaterals or the nervous system, working to prevent and cure diseases. If applied properly the different massage methods, though simple, can yield remarkable results.

During massage, attention should be paid to the method and force applied. There are many techniques of acupoint massage, with pressing, pushing and kneading being among the common ones.

1. Pressing

Method: Pressing refers to massage of a certain part of the body with a finger, palm, elbow or foot. It can reach as shallow as the muscle or as deep as the bone, joint or internal organ according to the force of pressure applied. The direction of the pressing should be vertical and the force should proceed from light to heavy. Relax the point after the pressure is held for some time or the force can be exerted continually. Pressing should be rhythmical and sudden application of force is contraindicated.

Function: To channel meridians and collaterals, open congestion, get rid of cold and stop pain, among others.

Variations: Acupoint massage via pressing is divided into finger pressing, palm pressing, elbow pressing and stamping.

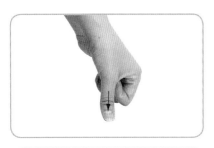

Finger pressing: This is the most common technique, with pressure applied by the pad of the thumb. The force of such pressing is determined by the tightness and tingling in the part concerned.

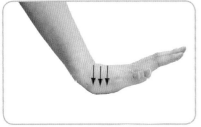

Palm pressing: Using the palm center or the heel of the palm, it is mostly used for larger body parts such as the waist, back or abdomen.

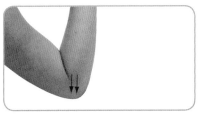

Elbow pressing: Using the point of the bent elbow, it is mostly applied to the deep layers or the acupoints of fleshy soft tissues such as the waist, buttocks or Huantiao point.

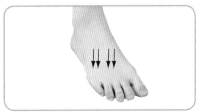

Stamping: This involves pressing with the foot, and it is often applied to such parts as the waist, buttocks and thighs.

2. Rubbing and Kneading

Method: Using the pad of the finger, palm heel or surface, or the thenar eminence, it focuses on the acupoint, rubbing and kneading gently around it. It differs from pressing as there is movement rather than a focus on one single spot.

Function: Beneficial for the body's vital energy and blood, energizing the blood, getting rid of dampness, and warming up meridians and collaterals among other effects.

Variations: These consist of finger rubbing and kneading, palm heel rubbing and kneading, and rubbing and kneading with the thenar eminence.

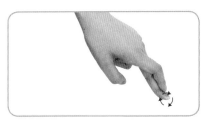

Finger rubbing and kneading: Using the pad of the thumb, the index finger or the middle finger, it is applied to acupoints on the body surface.

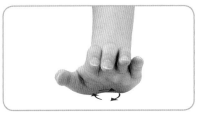

Palm heel rubbing and kneading: Using the palm heel, it is applied to the waist, abdomen and limbs, among other parts.

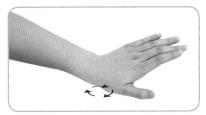

Rubbing and kneading with the thenar eminence: Using the thenar eminence, it is applied to the body surface.

Location of Thenar Eminence and Hypothenar Eminence

Thenar eminence. The fleshy part below the base of the thumb on the palm side, its muscles protrude prominently when the palm is stretched

Hypothenar eminence: Also on the palm side, between the small (pinky) finger and the wrist.

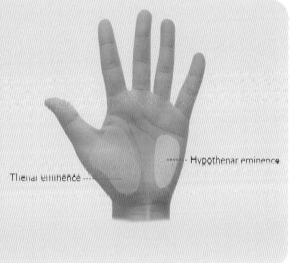

Hypothenar eminence

Thenar eminence

3. Massaging

Method: The palm or the finger pad is placed over the acupoint. Create force from the wrist and forearm, move in a rhythmic, circular, slow and gentle way.

Function: Beneficial for the spleen and stomach, smoothing qi and adjusting vital energy and blood, among others.

Variations: These consist of finger massage, palm massage and palm heel massage.

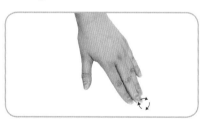

Finger massage: Keeping the wrist straight, the pad of the index, middle or ring finger is applied to a body part, circling around rhythmically. This technique is often used around the eyes.

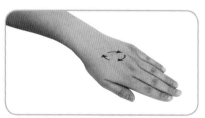

Palm massage: Keeping the wrist straight, the palm surface is applied to a body part, circling around rhythmically. This technique is often used on the abdomen.

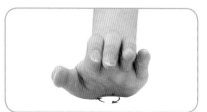

Palm heel massage: With the wrist bent, the thenar eminence and the hypothenar eminence of the palm heel are applied, with each finger slightly bent as well. It is often used on the head, back, waist and buttocks.

4. Clutching

Method: The thumb is coupled with either the middle or index finger, or all four fingers in an arc shape, to grab and press both sides of the acupoint symmetrically using soft and hard force alternately. It is often used on acupoints of the arms and legs.

Function: To channel meridians and collaterals, adjust yin and yang, get rid of the cold, dispel heat and stop pain, among others.

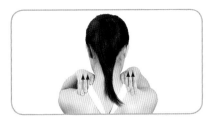

Clutching: The movement should be slow, gentle and continuous, rather than using sudden force.

5. Rubbing

Method: The palm, or the thenar eminence and the hypothenar eminence, or four closed fingers, are applied to a body part to rub back and forth in a linear way, producing considerable warmth.

Function: To benefit qi and blood, vitalize blood and channel collaterals, clear the chest, dispel liver congestion, get rid of dampness, warm up meridians and dispel cold.

Variations: There are three kinds: palm rubbing, thenar eminence rubbing and side rubbing.

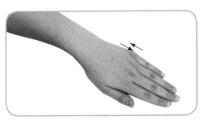

Palm rubbing: The surface of the straightened palm is applied closely to the skin, rubbing up and down, or left and right, or back and forth continuously. This massage is well suited to a large and flat area, such as the shoulders, back, chest or abdomen.

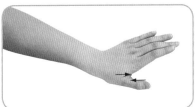

Thenar eminence rubbing: With the four fingers next to one another and slightly bent, the thenar eminence and palm heel are applied to the skin to rub back and forth in a linear way. This massage is suitable for smaller parts, such as four limbs.

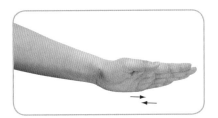

Side rubbing: The hypothenar eminence of the straightened palm is applied to the skin to rub back and forth in a linear way. This massage is suitable for the shoulders, back, waist and legs.

6. Pushing

Method: One of the most common techniques, pushing has many variations and uses.

Function: To channel qi, vitalize blood, eliminate convulsion and stop pain.

Variations: There are two common methods: finger pushing and palm pushing.

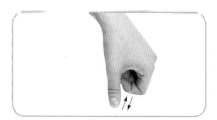

Finger pushing: With the straightened wrist joint as the center of force, the thumb tip is forcefully applied to the acupoint, moving back and forth rhythmically. It is mostly used for the head and abdomen.

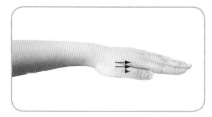

Palm pushing: One or both palms are applied to the skin to push and squeeze the muscle forward.

7. Pinching

Method: The nail of the thumb or index finger is used to forcefully pierce the acupoint. Pinching is often used in conjunction with kneading on the face and fingertips.

Function: To channel meridians, calm the mind, and bring mental clarity.

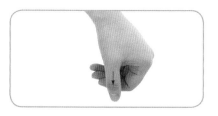

Single-hand pinching: The force of pinching increases gradually. Be mindful not to break the skin. The acupoint should be kneaded gently after pinching to ease discomfort.

8. Forceful Pointing

Method: The fingertip or the tip of a tool is applied with force. It is suitable for acupoints on the limbs, waist, back and buttocks.

Function: To channel meridians, get rid of the cold, and open up congestion.

Variations: This can be done with the thumb, with the knuckle or with three fingers.

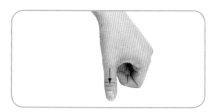

Forceful pointing with the thumb: The thumb tip, at an eighty-degree angle, is used to apply strong pressure at the acupoint.

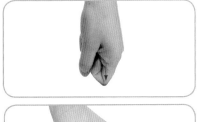

Forceful pointing with the knuckle: The tip of the knuckle is used to apply strong pressure at the acupoint.

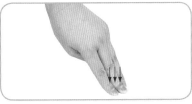

Forceful pointing with three fingers: The tips of the index, middle and ring finger are held next to one another, applying strong pressure at meridians and collaterals, without movement.

9. Twisting

Method: The pads of the thumb and index finger are used to hold the treated part, and then the fingers twist symmetrically with slight force. It is suitable for treatment of the fingers, back of the hand, and toes.

Function: To relax tendons, channel collaterals, smooth joints, and get rid of swelling and pain.

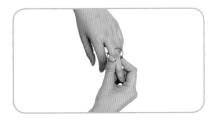

Twisting: The movement should be agile and rapid during the massage.

10. Pulling

Method: There are several combinations of fingers that may be used: the pads of the thumb and index finger, the thumb and the side of the second joint of the index finger, or the pads of the index and middle finger. The fingers grab and pull up the skin and then release immediately afterwards, making it produce sound. It is mostly applied to the forehead, and the rear and front of the neck and back.

Function: To reduce inner heat, channel skin, dispel harmful elements and get rid of the cold.

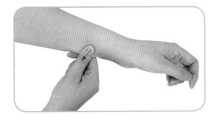

Pulling: Grab and pull up quickly and then suddenly release, until the treated part appears purple-red or bluish-red.

11. Clamping

Method: Two fingers clamp the treated part symmetrically, using considerable force to squeeze while moving gradually.

Function: To relax tendons and channel collaterals as well as vitalize qi and blood. Clamping serves to enhance skin and tendon movement as well as improve blood and lymph circulation.

Variation: There are three kinds: two-finger clamping, three-finger clamping and five-finger clamping. In addition either one or two hands can be used. Often two hands are used in massaging both sides of the spinal column, which is also called "the therapy of pinching the skin along the spinal column."

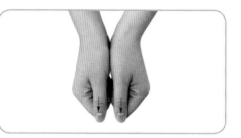

Two-finger clamping: The thumb and the radial margin of the middle section of the index finger are used to exert force.

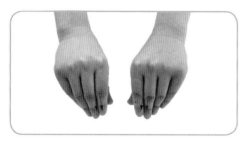

Three-finger clamping: The thumb, index finger and middle finger are used to exert force symmetrically.

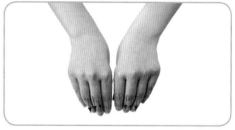

Five-finger clamping: In this variation the thumb and all the other fingers are used to exert force symmetrically.

Tips
- The surrounding should be quiet and clean with fresh air and appropriate temperature. Drafty places are undesirable.
- Before performing massage, fingernails must be trimmed and rings are not allowed.
- Hands should be kept clean and warm in order to avoid muscle tension or skin reactions. It is best to wash hands with warm water before massage.
- The patient should discharge urine and evacuate the bowels prior to treatment, and should wear suitable clothes.
- Remain calm, concentrated and light-hearted while massage is in progress.

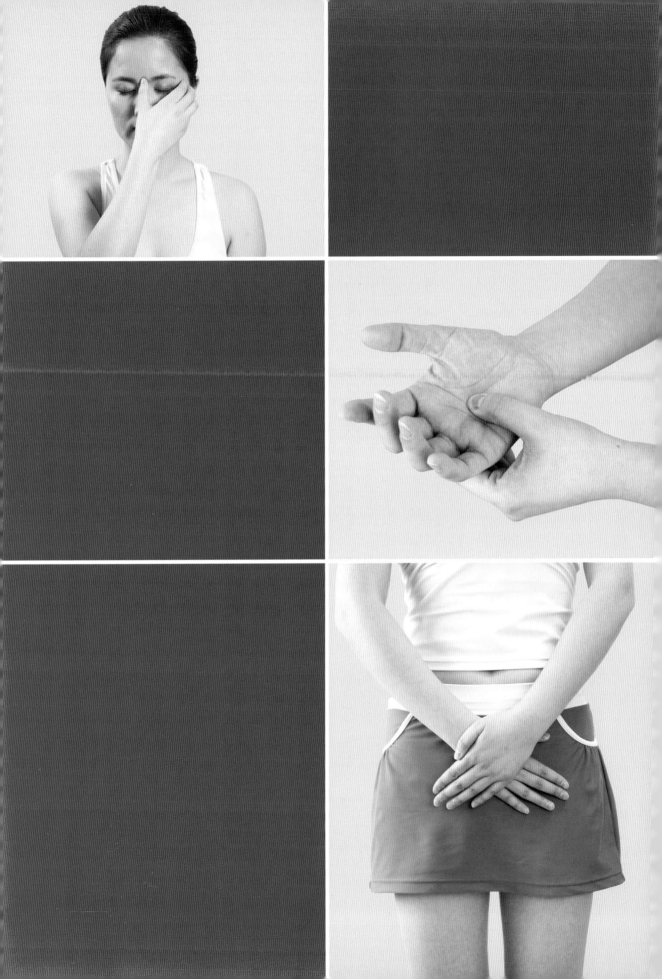

CHAPTER THREE
How to Find Acupoints Accurately

Massage acts chiefly as stimulation for acupoints as part of medical treatment and preventative healthcare. Therefore finding acupoints correctly is essential to effective massage. This book shows the general location of the acupoints, but it is important for you to practice finding them on your own.

Since ancient times in China, the position and measurement of acupoints have been described by the unit of the "body cun" (abbreviated as "cun" in this book). Acupoints are of different sizes and depths. This chapter gives an introduction to several simple and quick ways for accurately finding them.

1. Using Finger-Length Measurement

The finger length measurement of the body cun, a simple and convenient way to measure distance in locating acupoints, is based on the thumb width of the patient. With this highly individualized type of measurement, therefore, one cannot find the acupoints of another person according to one's own body cun, since this is not accurate.

Two Different Concepts: Cun and the Body Cun
- "Cun" is a traditional standard unit of length in China. One cun is about 3.33 centimeters.
- "Body cun" is a measurement specific to the individual, used as the unit of length for measuring acupoints.

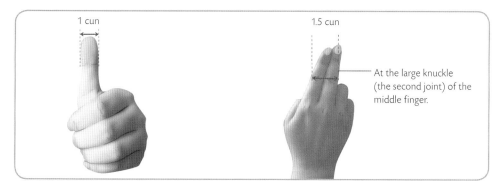

One cun. The width of the thumb joint of the patient.

One and a half cun: Measuring at the level of the large knuckle (the second joint) of the middle finger, the width of the index and middle finger closed together is 1.5 cun.

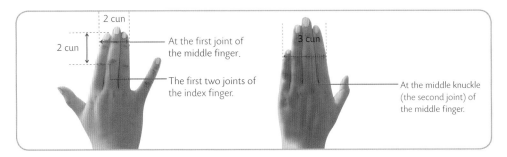

Two cun: With the index finger, middle and ring finger closed together, take the measurement at the level of the first joint of the middle finger. The length of the first two joints of the index finger is also two cun.

Three cun: With the four fingers closed, measure at the level of the large knuckle (the second joint) of the middle finger.

2. Using Bone-Length Measurement

To ascertain the location of acupoints we can also use the measurement between bone joints. (More about the names of bones can be found in the next section.) Measurement can be made according to corresponding bone-length for people of different sexes, ages, height and weight. For any individual, the vertical cun and horizontal cun are the same length; the difference in name relates solely to direction.

- Horizontal cun: Mostly applied to measuring the front and rear of the body, one measures acupoints on each side in relation to their distance from the front central line.
- Vertical cun: Mostly applied to measuring acupoints upward and downward, with joints used as the basis for measurement.

3. Using Physical Marks of the Body

Physical marks on human body, such as eyebrows, nipples and ankles can also serve as locators of acupoints.

- The eyes, nose, mouth, ears, eyebrows and hairline serve as marks on the head. For instance the Yintang point lies between the eyebrows.
- On the abdomen, the nipples, xiphoid process and navel serve as marks. For instance the Zhongwan point lies between the xiphoid process and navel, while the Danzhong point lies between the nipples.
- Joints and ankles serve as marks on four limbs. For instance, Yanglingquan point lies in the anterior inferior part of the fibular head.

4. Using Pressing

Most of the acupoints are in a cavity, which is the key to the positioning.

The patient will feel a sense of tingling, numbness, swelling and pain when the correct location of the acupoint is pressed.

5. Using Special Postures

You can also make use of some special postures to find acupoints. For instance the Quchi point lies at the end of a bent elbow. The Jiexi point can be found on the back of the foot when it is bent, between the two tendons bordering the heel and the lower leg. The Ququan point lies at the end of the bend of the knee.

Location	Starting and Ending Points	Cun	Measurement
Head and face	A: From middle of frontal hairline to middle of rear hairline.	12 cun	vertical cun
	B: From Yintang point to middle of frontal hairline.	3 cun	vertical cun
	C: From Dazhui point to middle of rear hairline.	3 cun	vertical cun
	D: From Yintang point to Dazhui point.	18 cun	vertical cun
	E: Between two Touwei points on forehead.	9 cun	horizontal cun
	F: Between two mastoids (Wangu points) behind ears.	9 cun	horizontal cun
Chest and abdomen	G: From Tiantu point to bottom of sternum.	9 cun	vertical cun
	H: From bottom of sternum to Qizhong point.	8 cun	vertical cun
	I: From Qizhong point to Qugu point.	5 cun	vertical cun
	J: Between two nipples.	8 cun	horizontal cun
	K: From top of armpit to Zhangmen point.	12 cun	vertical cun
Back	L: From margo medialis of scapula to posterior midline.	3 cun	horizontal cun
Arms	M: From frontal crease and rear crease of armpit to cubital crease (inside of elbow).	9 cun	vertical cun
	N: From inside of elbow to side bend of wrist.	12 cun	vertical cun
Legs	O: From upper margin of pubic bone to upper margin of epicondyle of femur.	18 cun	vertical cun
	P: From lower margin of condylus medialis tibiae to inner ankle tip.	13 cun	vertical cun
	Q: From greater trochanter of femur to bend at back of knee.	19 cun	vertical cun
	R: From bend at back of knee to outer ankle tip.	16 cun	vertical cun

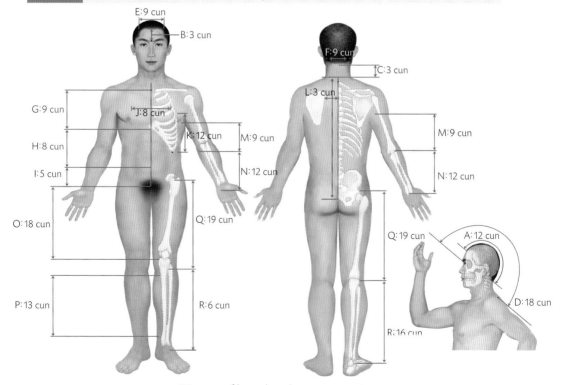

Diagram of bone-length measurement.

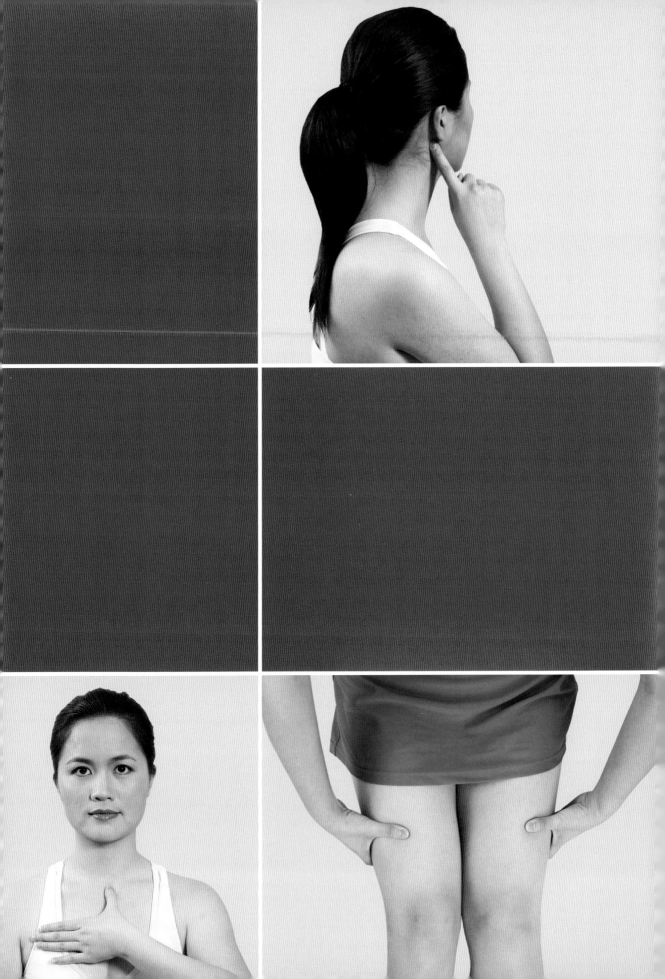

CHAPTER FOUR
Acupoint Massage for Health and Beauty

1 | Migraine

The most common and important type of migraine is vascular migraine, which is marked by throbbing pain or distending pain corresponding to pulse. It is caused by dysfunction of the intracranial artery contraction and expansion. In relation to TCM treatment it is also called an angioneurotic headache.

Symptoms

In clinical practice, migraine is divided into three periods, i.e., the period of intracranial vascular contraction, the period of extracranial vascular expansion, and the period of alleviation. These three periods are inseparable and there is no obvious interval. The length of each period varies with the individual and some people may show no preclinical (intracranial) phase.

• Period of intracranial vascular contraction: Also called the preclinical phase, it generally takes place several minutes or even an hour before the headache attacks. It is chiefly marked by the lack of blood supply to the brain, which may manifest as seeing stars, compromised or lost vision, short-term numbness of one side of the body, limb weakness or unclear verbal expression. However it rarely develops into permanent harm. These symptoms foretell the imminent onset of headache.

• Period of extracranial vascular expansion: Headaches caused by vascular expansion generally last for several hours or days. Such headaches may be marked by continuous throbbing pain, dull pain or distending pain in one side or both sides of the temple. Most of the symptoms are severe, to the extent of affecting work and study. They may be accompanied by weakness all over the body, pale or red face, agitation, nausea, vomiting, loss of appetite and palpitations. The headache may be alleviated or eliminated when the patient falls asleep.

• Period of alleviation: The vascular expansion and headache will gradually return to normal after a period of time. In this period all the symptoms mentioned above disappear. The patients feel normal, except a few who suffer from insomnia, weakness and a lot of dreams in sleep. This period may last for several weeks or even months.

Target Acupoints

Head and neck: Baihui (DU 20), Touwei (ST 8), Taiyang (EX-HN 5), Shuaigu (GB 8), Qiangjian (DU 18), Fengchi (GB 20), Tianzhu (BL 10), Yifeng (SJ 17).

Arms: Waiguan (SJ 5), Yangxi (LI 5).

Legs: Yanglingquan (GB 34), Taichong (LV 3), Sanyinjiao (SP 6), Taibai (SP 3), Zutonggu (BL 66).

Recommended Massage

1. Pressing and Kneading the Touwei Point

Location: Front of the head at the hairline, 0.5 cun from the center line on both sides.

Method: Sit upright or lie on the back. Use the pad of the middle finger to rub and knead the Touwei point on both sides of the head. Continue for about two minutes and then press for 30 seconds, ideally until you feel the tingling and expansion radiate to the entire front of the head and both sides of the point.

Effect: Cure itchy scalp, migraine, forehead neuralgia, high blood pressure, conjunctivitis, decline of eyesight, and eye tearing.

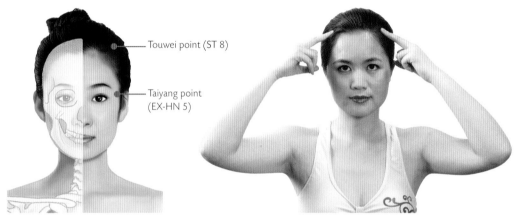

Touwei point (ST 8)

Taiyang point (EX-HN 5)

Location of the Touwei and Taiyang points.   Press and knead the Touwei point.

2. Pressing and Kneading the Taiyang Point

Location: In the depression about one cun behind the space between the outer tip of the brow and outer eye corner.

Method: Sit upright or lie on the back. Use the pad of the index finger to press the Taiyang points on both sides of the head, rubbing and kneading for two minutes until you feel tingling and expansion in the acupoints. If rubbing and kneading of a larger area is required, or you need more force, use the thenar eminences.

Effect: Cure cold, headache, fever, dizziness, and red and swollen eyes with pain.

3. Rubbing and Kneading the Baihui Point

Location: At the center of the skull directly on top of the head, over the two ear tips.

Method: Sit upright or lie on the back. Use the middle or index finger to rub and knead for two minutes. Then press the Baihui point for 30 seconds, ideally until you feel the tingling and expansion radiate to the entire head.

Effect: Cure headache, migraine, dizziness, baldness, panic, forgetfulness, high blood pressure, low blood pressure, apoplexy, tinnitus, insomnia, nasal congestion, proctoptosis, hemorrhoids (piles) and diarrhea.

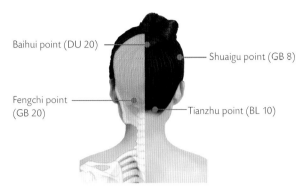

Baihui point (DU 20)

Shuaigu point (GB 8)

Fengchi point
(GB 20)

Tianzhu point (BL 10)

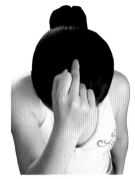

Location of the Baihui, Shuaigu, Fengchi and Tianzhu points.

Rub and knead the Baihui point.

4. Pressing and Kneading the Shuaigu Point

Location: On the side of the head, four centimeters above the tip of the ear.

Method: Sit upright or lie on the back. Use the index or middle finger to rub and knead the Shuaigu point on both sides for about two minutes until you feel tingling and expansion on both sides of the head.

Effect: Cure migraine, dizziness, vomiting and unhealthy hair.

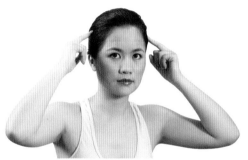

Press and knead the Shuaigu point.

5. Pressing and Kneading the Fengchi Point

Location: In the depression on both sides of the large tendon behind the nape of the neck, next to the lower edge of the skull.

Method: Sit upright. Place the thumb pads on the Fengchi point on either side of the head, with the remaining fingers holding the head. Press, rub and knead for two minutes proceeding from light to heavy force. Then press the Fengchi point for another 30 seconds, until you feel tingling and distension in the related part.

Effect: Cure migraine, headache with distension, dizziness, seeing stars, facial heat, tinnitus, fever, neck pain, red and swollen eyes with pain.

6. Pressing the Tianzhu Point

Location: At the rear of the head, 1.5 cun from the middle line and one cun above the hairline.

Method: Using the thumb, press the Tianzhu point of the same side of the head. As the head turns to the other side, the thumb should press downwards on the Tianzhu point in a slanting manner.

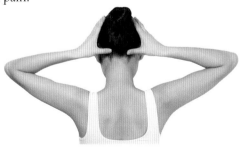

Press the Tianzhu point.

Effect: Get rid of cold, tranquilize the spirit, and cure fever, dizziness, neck-shoulder tingling and pain, cervical spondylosis, drowsiness, fatigue, low blood pressure, high blood pressure, drunkenness and car sickness.

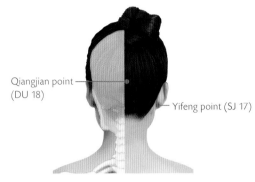

Qiangjian point (DU 18)

Yifeng point (SJ 17)

Location of the Qiangjian and Yifeng points.

7. Pressing and Kneading the Qiangjian Point

Location: In the middle of the back of the head, four cun above the rear hairline.

Method: Sitting upright, use the thumb or middle finger to press the Qiangjian point for 30 seconds. Then press, rub and knead for two minutes until you feel tingling and distension as the best effect.

Effect: Cure headache, dizziness, neck pain, epilepsy, agitation and insomnia.

8. Pressing and Kneading the Yifeng Point

Location: Behind the earlobe in a notch between the mastoid process and the lower frontal angle.

Method: Place the tip of the index or middle finger on the Yifeng point, pressing and then rubbing and kneading, moving from light to heavy force. Usually pressing lasts for 30 seconds, followed by rubbing and kneading for two minutes until you feel tingling and distension at the Yifeng point. Ideally this feeling will radiate to the inner ears.

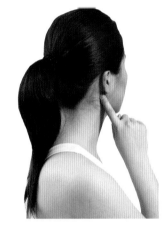

Press and knead the Yifeng point.

Effect: Cure deafness, tinnitus, dumbness, facioplegia, facial convulsion, trifacial neuralgia, tympanitis, external otitis (ear infection), tonsil inflammation, mandibular arthritis, stomatitis, hypertrophy of thyroid glands, toothache, eye disease, migraine and phrenospasm (spasm of the diaphragm).

9. Pressing the Waiguan and Neiguan Points

Location: The Waiguan point is in the middle on the outside of the arm, between the ulna and radius about two cun away from the horizontal line of the wrist joint. The Neiguan point is between the two tendons about two cun above the wrist joint bend.

Method: With the front arm bent halfway, use one thumb tip to press the Waiguan point on the other arm. The index or middle finger should press the Neiguan

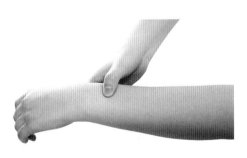

Press the Waiguan and Neiguan points.

point, pressing inward 20 to 30 times, until tingling and distension are felt.

Effect: Cure fever, cold, pneumonia, tinnitus, dumbness, stiff neck, migraine, intercostal nerve pain, upper limb joint pain, and elbow pain.

10. Pressing and Kneading the Yangxi Point

Location: At the wrist on the thumb side in a notch between two strained tendons when the thumb tilts upward.

Method: With the front arm bent halfway, use one thumb pad to press the Yangxi point of the other hand. Press, rub and knead for two to three minutes until tingling and distension are felt in the part concerned.

Effect: Cure wrist joint pain, peritendinitis, problems with the wrist joints and surrounding soft tissues, front arm pain, paralysis of one side of the body, headache, red and swollen eyes with pain and deafness.

11. Pinching the Yanglingquan Point

Location: On the outer side of the shin in a notch at the front lower part of the fibula.

Method: Sit upright. Use the thumb tip to pinch the Yanglingquan point forcefully, with pressure directed toward the toes for about one minute, until obvious tingling and distension are felt as the best effect.

Effect: Cure migraine, dizziness, red face, red eyes, sore throat, toothache, acne, hives, erysipelas and arm pain.

12. Pressing and Kneading the Taichong Point

Location: On the foot in a notch between the first and second metatarsal bones.

Method: Sit upright. Use the thumb tip to press, rub and knead the Taichong point for about two minutes and then press for another 30 seconds until tingling and

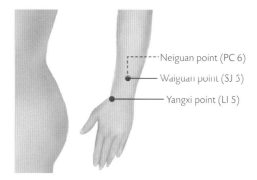

Location of the Neiguan, Waiguan and Yangxi points.

Neiguan point (PC 6)
Waiguan point (SJ 5)
Yangxi point (LI 5)

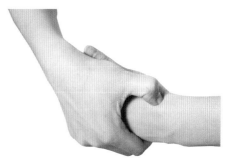

Press and knead the Yangxi point.

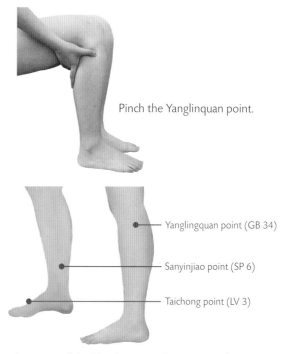

Pinch the Yanglinquan point.

Yanglingquan point (GB 34)

Sanyinjiao point (SP 6)

Taichong point (LV 3)

Location of the Yanglingquan, Sanyinjiao and Taichong points.

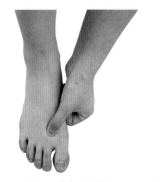

Press and knead the Taichong point.

distension are felt in the part concerned as the best effect.

Effect: Cure headache with distension, dizziness, migraine, menstrual disorder including dysmenorrhea and amenorrhea, and breast pain with distension.

13. Pressing and Kneading the Sanyinjiao Point

Location: At the rear edge of the shinbone, three cun above the ankle.

Method: Sit upright and place one shin on the opposite thigh. Use the thumb to press, rub and knead the Sanyinjiao point for about two minutes until tingling and distension are felt in the part concerned as the best effect.

Effect: Cure insomnia, palpitation, high blood pressure, menstrual disorder, dysmenorrhea, impotence and nocturnal emission.

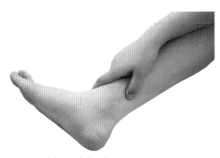

Press and knead the Sanyinjiao point.

14. Pressing the Taibai Point

Location: On the inside of the foot, near the ball of the foot at the first metatarsophalangeal joint.

Method: Sit upright, with one leg extended out to the floor, and the opposite leg placed on the knee of this extended leg. Use the thumb to press the Taibai point for about ten minutes continuously each time until tingling and distension are felt as the best effect.

Effect: Chiefly serve to cure stomachalgia, abdominal distension, vomiting, hiccups, borborygmus, diarrhea, dysentery, constipation, dermatophytosis and anal fistula.

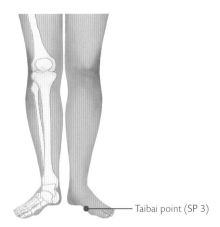

Taibai point (SP 3)

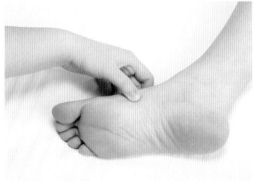

Press the Taibai point.

15. Pressing and Kneading the Zutonggu Point

Location: Along the outer side of the foot, at the border of the sole (which will be marked by a change to lighter skin in many people), at the far end of the fifth metatarsophalangeal joint.

Method: Sit with crossed legs. Hold one knee while using the thumb to press the Zutonggu point of the same side. Bend the finger joint into a ninety-degree angle to press, rub and knead a small area in a circular manner.

Effect: Chiefly serve to cure headache, stiff neck, dizziness, nose bleeding and epilepsy.

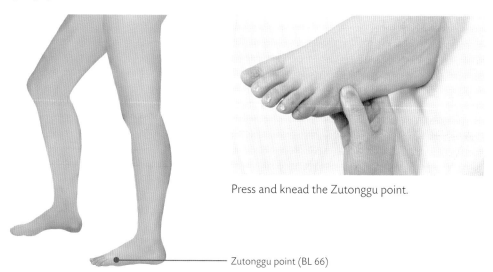

Press and knead the Zutonggu point.

Zutonggu point (BL 66)

Tips

Climatic changes, diet and medicine may contribute to the onset of migraines. Therefore attention should be paid to eliminating or reducing the causes.
• Avoid red wine and cheese.
• Avoid overwork and agitation while ensuring enough sleep.
• Note that headaches may be related to problems with eyes, ears, nose, paranasal sinus, teeth and neck. Pay attention to preventing infection. Priority should be given to treating tooth problems.
    Migraine attacks may be alleviated by the following methods; please note that timely diagnosis and medical treatment are required if the case becomes serious.
• Use an ice bag for cold compression.
• Coil the head with a towel.
• Lie down and rest.
• Drink green tea.
• Meditate.

2 Facial Paralysis

This common ailment is primarily marked by functional inhibition of muscular movements relating to facial expression. It is not limited by age or sex.

In these cases acupuncture and moxibustion are not recommended. Despite displaying very good curative effect for other diseases, they are not necessarily suitable for facial paralysis (facioplegia). For many patients with facial paralysis, undergoing acupuncture and moxibustion in the early stage may cause aftereffects, leading to great difficulties in later treatment.

Symptoms

With most cases of facial paralysis, patients suddenly find that one side of the cheek feels inactive and the mouth corner pulls upward when washing the face and rinsing the mouth in early morning.

As for patients with complete paralysis of facial expression, they are marked by the disappearance of forehead wrinkles, expansion of the palpebral fissure, and flatness of the nasolabial grooves, with drooping mouth corner on the affected side, and tooth exposure and an upward-pulling mouth corner toward the sound side.

The patient cannot furrow the forehead and brows, close the eyes, or puff out or pout the mouth. They cannot fully close the mouth when puffing out cheeks or whistling. While eating, food residues often stay behind between the teeth and the cheek of the affected side, often with saliva dripping. Tears cannot fall normally since the lower eyelids turn inward.

Target Acupoints

Head and neck: Yuyao (EX-HN 4), Jingming (BL 1), Chengqi (ST 1), Quanliao (SI 18), Yingxiang (LI 20), Jiache (ST 6), Dicang (ST 4), Chengjiang (SP 24), Cuanzhu (BL 2), Yifeng (SJ 17).
Arms: Hegu (LI 4).
Legs: Taichong (LV 3).

Recommended Massage

1. Pressing and Kneading the Yuyao Point
Location: Directly above the pupil in the middle of each eyebrow.

Method: Use the pads of the two index or middle fingers to gently press and knead the Yuyao points above the eyes for two minutes, until tingling and distension are felt as the best effect.

Effect: Cure forehead pain, drooping eyelids, red and swollen eyes with pain, slight corneal opacity and myopia.

2. Pressing and Kneading the Jingming Point

Location: In the depression over the inner corner of the eye.

Method: Lie on the back or sit upright. Use the thumb tip, index finger or middle finger to press the Jingming point of the affected side, pressing the inner upper part for two minutes until some tingling and distension are felt as the best effect.

Effect: Ease fatigue and restore eyesight, as well as treat bloodshot eyes, red swelling, edema, glaucoma and cataract. In addition it can ease nasal congestion when accompanied by massage of acupoints around the nose.

3. Pressing and Kneading the Chengqi Point

Location: Directly below the pupil, between the lower edge of the eyeball and the eye socket.

Method: Lie on the back or sit upright. Use the pad of the index finger to press and knead the margin in the middle of the suborbital part of the affected side. Continue for two minutes, until some tingling and distension are felt as the best effect.

Effect: Treat acute and chronic conjunctivitis, myopia, astigmatism, glaucoma, early-stage cataract, optic nerve atrophy, ceratitis, retinitis pigmentosa, eyelid spasm and diabetes insipidus.

4. Pressing and Kneading the Quanliao Point

Location: Directly in the lower part of the outer canthus, in a cavity of the lower margin of the cheekbone.

Method: Lie on the back or sit upright. Use the index or middle finger to press and knead the Quanliao point of the affected side for about 30 seconds. Then continue for two minutes, until some tingling and distension are felt in the part concerned and radiated to the entire face as

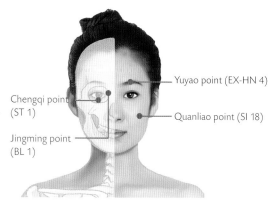

Location of the Yuyao, Chengqi, Quanliao and Jingming points.

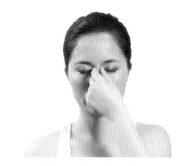

Press and knead the Jingming point.

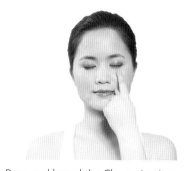

Press and knead the Chengqi point.

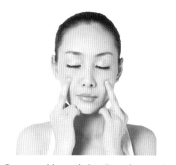

Press and knead the Quanliao point.

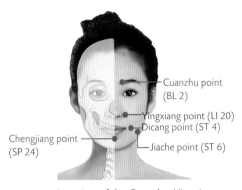

Cuanzhu point (BL 2)

Yingxiang point (LI 20)
Dicang point (ST 4)

Chengjiang point (SP 24)

Jiache point (ST 6)

Location of the Cuanzhu, Yingxiang, Dicang, Chengjiang and Jiache points.

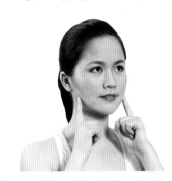

Press and knead the Jiache point.

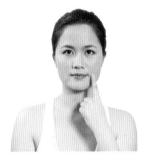

Press and knead the Dicang point.

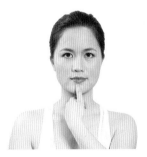

Press and knead the Chengjiang point.

the best effect.

Effect: Chiefly serve to treat toothache, trifacial neuralgia, mandibular arthritis, dislocation of lower jaw, convulsion of the zygomaxillary muscle, facial convulsion, facioplegia, tympanitis, dizziness and tinnitus.

5. Pressing and Kneading the Jiache Point

Location: In a cavity about one cun in the upper part of the lower jaw corner, i.e. the highest point of the zygomaxillary muscle when one chews.

Method: Lie on the back or sit upright. Use the index finger to press and knead the Jiache point on the affected side for about two minutes, or press and knead it until you feel the secretion of fluid in the mouth.

Effect: Treat maxillary division or mandibular division pain of the trigeminal nerve, problems with the zygomaxillary muscle, difficulty in opening the mouth, toothache, facioplegia, deviated mouth and eyes (due to facial paralysis), salivating, freckles and chloasma.

6. Pressing and Kneading the Dicang Point

Location: About 0.4 cun away from the mouth corner, directly in line with the pupil.

Method: Lie on the back or sit upright. Use the index finger to gently press and knead the Dicang point on the affected side for about two minutes until some tingling and distension are felt as the best effect.

Effect: Treat facioplegia, facial convulsion, trifacial neuralgia, mouth and lip edema, mouth and lip herpes, excessive salivation in children, angular stomatitis, toothache, gingivitis and oral ulcer.

7. Pushing and Kneading the Chengjiang Point

Location: Right in a cavity in the center directly below the lower lip.

Method: Use the thumb tip to press and knead the Chengjiang point for two minutes and then push to the mouth corner toward the Dicang point of the affected part. Knead and press for a short while. Knead further along the upper lip to the Renzhong point, back and forth, 15 or 20 times, until some tingling and distension are felt as the best effect.

Effect: Cure and prevent facial convulsion, facial neuritis, gingivitis, stomatitis, mouth and lip furuncle (skin abscess) and angular stomatitis.

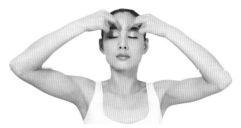

Press and knead the Cuanzhu point.

8. Pressing and Kneading the Cuanzhu Point

Location: In a cavity where the inner eyebrow starts.

Method: Use the pad of the middle finger to press the Cuanzhu point on the affected side. When there is a sense of tingling and distension, gradually increase force until tingling and distension radiate to the eyes, pressing for about two minutes in total.

Effect: It has a very good effect on eye tearing, dizziness, visual fatigue, eye edema, conjunctivitis, cheek pain, headache and high blood pressure. The Cuanzhu point is also often used in facial beauty treatment.

9. Pressing and Kneading the Yingxiang Point

Location: Beside the wing of the nose, 0.5 cun away, in the nasolabial groove.

Method: Sitting upright, first use the index finger to press and knead the point for two minutes and then press for another 30 seconds, until some tingling and distension are felt as the best effect.

Effect: Excellent for easing various symptoms involving the nose, such as runny nose, nasal congestion, nose bleeding, nasosinusitis, decline of sense of smell, and chronic rhinitis. In addition this acupoint is also frequently used in cases of trifacial neuralgia and to treat the aftereffect of facial paralysis, as well as for facial beauty.

10. Pinching and Kneading the Hegu Point

Location: In the highest point on the back of the hand between the thumb base and the base of the index finger (in the webbing between these two fingers).

Method: Use the thumb tip of one hand to pinch the Hegu point on the other hand for about one minute, and continue pinching and kneading for about two minutes, until some tingling and distension are felt as the best effect.

Effect: Treat facioplegia, trigeminal pain, facial paralysis, deviated mouth and eyes (facial paralysis), rhinitis, headache, toothache, acne, visual fatigue, sore throat, tinnitus and hiccups.

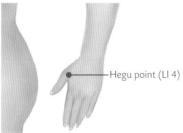

Hegu point (LI 4)

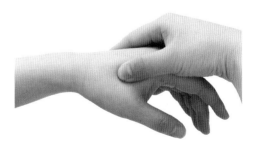

Pinch and knead the Hegu point.

11. Pressing and Kneading the Yifeng Point

Location: Behind the earlobe in a notch between the mastoid process and the lower frontal angle.

Method: Place the tip of the index or middle finger on the Yifeng point, pressing and then rubbing and kneading, moving from light to heavy force. Usually pressing lasts for 30 seconds, followed by rubbing and kneading for two minutes until you feel tingling and distension at the Yifeng point. Ideally this feeling will radiate to the inner ears.

Effect: Cure deafness, tinnitus, dumbness, facioplegia, facial convulsion, trifacial neuralgia, tympanitis, external otitis (ear infection), tonsil inflammation, mandibular arthritis, stomatitis, hypertrophy of thyroid glands, toothache, eye disease, migraine and phrenospasm (spasm of the diaphragm).

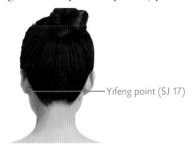
Yifeng point (SJ 17)

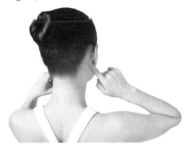

Press and knead the Yifeng point.

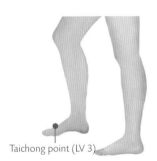
Taichong point (LV 3)

Location of the Taichong point.

12. Pressing and Kneading the Taichong Point

Location: On the foot in a notch between the first and second metatarsal bones.

Method: Sit upright. Use the thumb tip to press, rub and knead the Taichong point for about two minutes and then press for another 30 seconds until tingling and distension are felt in the part concerned as the best effect.

Effect: Cure headache with distension, dizziness, migraine, menstrual disorder including dysmenorrhea and amenorrhea, and breast pain with distension.

Tips

- Keep warm and avoid direct exposure to cold wind on the face. The following people should be particularly mindful to avoid walking in draft: the old, weak, those recovering from illness or after drinking, and patients suffering from high blood pressure, arthritis and other chronic diseases.
- Those in a weakened condition should make active efforts to strengthen their physique in order to reinforce resistance against illness. This includes eating more fruits and vegetables. Particularly at the change of seasons, they are advised to eat more Chinese leeks, celery, spring bamboo-shoots and mustards, which not only strengthen the body but also increase resistance against illness.

3 Facial Convulsion

This refers to paroxysmal, uncontrolled and irregular muscular twitch, without other kinds of symptoms related to damage of the nervous system. Facial convulsion is mostly caused by the aftereffect of neuritis but the pathogeny is not clear.

Symptoms

Twitching is seldom seen on both sides of the face. Patients are mostly women. Spasmodic and light twitching of the orbicularis oculi muscle on the lower eyelid is often seen, gradually spreading to one side of the face, with mouth corner twitching being the most obvious manifestation.

The extent of twitch can vary. It will become serious when the patient is nervous, excited or tired, and these symptoms may disappear when the patient is quiet or falls asleep. For a few patients, facial twitching may affect the facial muscles of one entire side of the face.

Target Acupoints

Head and neck: Yintang (EX-HN 3), Taiyang (EX-HN 5), Chengqi (ST 1), Dicang (ST 4), Renzhong (DU 26), Sibai (ST 2), Fengchi (GB 20), Xiaguan (ST 7), Jiache (ST 6), Tongziliao (GB 1).
Arms: Hegu (LI 4).

Recommended Massage

1. Pressing and Kneading the Yintang Point

Location: At the central point right between the eyebrows.

Method: Lie on the back or sit upright. Use the pad of the index finger to press and knead the Yintang point for two minutes and then continue for another 30 seconds until tingling and distension are felt as the best effect.

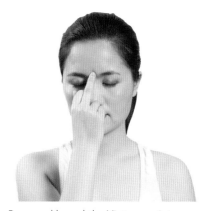

Press and knead the Yintang point.

Effect: Treat cold, vascular headache, frontal sinusitis, supra-orbital neuralgia, acute and chronic rhinitis, nose bleeding, nasal polyp, high blood pressure, neurasthenia, malaria, nervous vomiting, postpartum anemic fainting, eclampsia, febrile convulsion, facial convulsion, facioplegia, acute and chronic conjunctivitis.

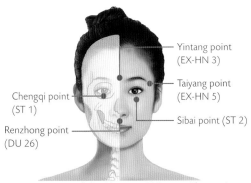

Location of the Yintang, Taiyang, Chengqi, Sibai and Renzhong points.

Yintang point (EX-HN 3)

Taiyang point (EX-HN 5)

Chengqi point (ST 1)

Sibai point (ST 2)

Renzhong point (DU 26)

2. Pressing and Kneading the Taiyang Point

Location: In the depression about one cun behind the space between the outer tip of the brow and outer eye corner.

Method: Use the pad of both thumbs to press and knead the Taiyang point on both sides of the head respectively for two minutes, until some tingling and distension are felt as the best effect. If working on a larger area or if heavier force is needed to press and knead, use the thenar eminences.

Effect: Treat cold, fever, headache, dizziness, red and swollen eyes with pain.

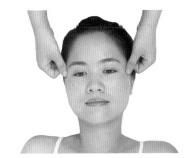

Press and knead the Taiyang point.

3. Pressing and Kneading the Chengqi Point

Location: Directly below the pupil, between the lower edge of the eyeball and the eye socket.

Method: Lie on the back or sit upright. Use the pad of the middle finger to press and knead the point on the affected side for two minutes, until some tingling and distension are felt as the best effect.

Effect: Treat acute and chronic conjunctivitis, myopia, astigmatism, glaucoma, early-stage cataract, optic nerve atrophy, ceratitis, retinitis pigmentosa, eyelid spasm and diabetes insipidus.

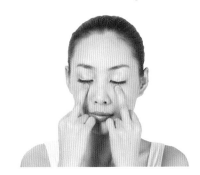

Press and knead the Chengqi point.

4. Pinching and Kneading the Renzhong Point

Location: In the middle of the groove below the nose, between the lip and the nose.

Method: Lie on the back or sit upright. Use the thumb tip to pinch the Renzhong point for about one minute. Then press and knead it for another two minutes, until some tingling and distension are felt as the best effect.

Effect: Treat unconsciousness, fainting, nasal congestion, lumbar sprain and facial paralysis.

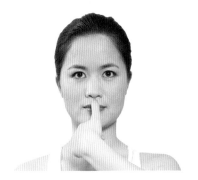

Press and knead the Renzhong point.

5. Pressing and Kneading the Sibai Point
Location: Directly below the pupil, in a cavity below the orbit.

Method: Use the pads of the middle fingers to press the Sibai point on both sides. When there is tingling and pain, gradually increase force, pressing and kneading for about two minutes, so that the radiating tingling and distension reaches to the eyes.

Effect: It has a very good effect on symptoms caused by facioplegia such as failure to open and close the eyes, pain near the cheeks, trigeminal pain, myopia, visual fatigue and giddiness. In addition it is also an acupoint frequently used in facial beauty therapy.

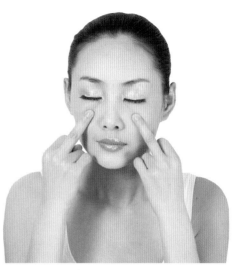
Press and knead the Sibai point.

6. Pressing and Kneading the Fengchi Point
Location: In the depression on both sides of the large tendon behind the nape of the neck, next to the lower edge of the skull.

Method: Use the pad of the index and middle fingers to press and knead the Fengchi point on both sides for two minutes, proceeding from light to heavy force, until some tingling and distension are felt as the best effect.

Effect: Treat cold, fever, neck pain, headache, dizziness, and red and swollen eyes with pain.

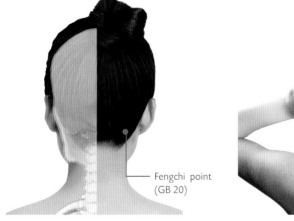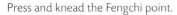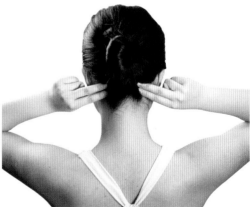

Fengchi point (GB 20)

Press and knead the Fengchi point.

7. Pressing and Kneading the Xiaguan Point
Location: In the depression at the hairline in front of the ear; it can be felt when the mouth is closed and creases when the mouth is open.

Method: Lie on the back or sit upright. Use the middle finger to press and

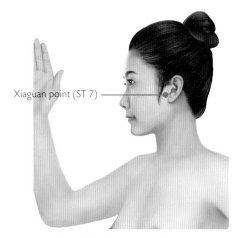

Xiaguan point (ST 7)

Location of the Xiaguan point.

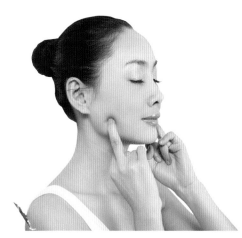

Press and knead the Jiache point.

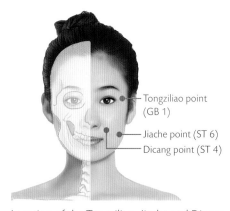

Tongziliao point (GB 1)

Jiache point (ST 6)

Dicang point (ST 4)

Location of the Tongziliao, Jiache and Dicang points.

knead the Xiaguan point of the affected side for two minutes. Then continue for another 30 seconds, until some tingling and distension are felt, ideally radiating all over the face.

Effect: Treat toothache, trifacial neuralgia, mandibular arthritis, dislocation of lower jaw joints, convulsion of the masseter, facial convulsion, facioplegia, tympanitis, deafness, dumbness, dizziness and tinnitus.

8. Pressing and Kneading the Jiache Point

Location: In a cavity about one cun in the upper part of the lower jaw corner, i.e. the highest point of the zygomaxillary muscle when one chews.

Method: Use the pad of the middle finger to press and knead the Jiache point of the affected side for about two minutes. Use moderate force until some tingling and distension are felt along with slight warmth and numbness as the best effect.

Effect: Treat toothache, trifacial neuralgia, problems with the masseter, difficulty in opening the mouth, freckles, chloasma, deviated mouth and eyes (facial paralysis), and excess salivating.

9. Pressing and Kneading the Tongziliao Point

Location: At the point 0.5 cun laterally outside of the outer canthus.

Method: Use the pad of the index finger to press the Tongziliao point of the affected side. When there is tingling and pain, increase force to press and knead for two minutes, radiating the tingling and distension to the eyes.

Effect: It has a very good effect on curing headache, dizziness, seeing stars, visual fatigue, eye itch and conjunctival congestion. It is also an important acupoint for eye beauty therapy.

10. Pressing and Kneading the Dicang Point

Location: About 0.4 cun away from the mouth corner, directly in line with the pupil.

Method: Lie on the back or sit upright. Use the index finger to gently press and knead the Dicang point on the affected side for about two minutes until some tingling and distension are felt as the best effect.

Effect: Treat facioplegia, facial convulsion, trifacial neuralgia, mouth and lip edema, mouth and lip herpes, excessive salivation in children, angular stomatitis, toothache, gingivitis and oral ulcer.

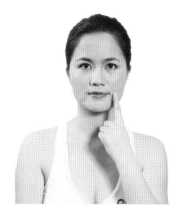

Press and knead the Dicang point.

11. Pinching and Kneading the Hegu Point

Location: In the highest point on the back of the hand between the thumb base and the base of the index finger (in the webbing between these two fingers).

Method: Use the thumb of one hand to press the Hegu point on the other hand; if the left side of the face is affected, the Hegu point on the right should be pinched and kneaded, and vice versa.

Effect: Treat cold, runny nose, headache, toothache, acne, visual fatigue, sore throat, tinnitus and hiccups.

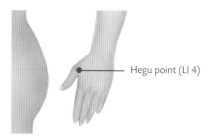

Hegu point (LI 4)

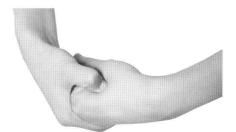

Pinch and knead the Hegu point.

Tips

Patients affected by facial convulsions are advised to adopt the following habits:
- Eat nutritious foods such as fresh fruits, vegetables, fish, beans and whole grains.
- Take sufficient B-type vitamins.
- Refrain from washing one's face with cold water, and pay attention to keeping the head and face warm.
- Avoid external irritation factors as well as UV rays while restricting computer and television use.

4 Facial Nerve Pain

Generally speaking, facial nerve pain refers to trigeminal neuralgia, which is marked by spasmodic sharp pain in the area of the trigeminal nerve. Facial nerve pain may be manifested in the forehead, scalp, eyes, nose, lips, cheeks, upper jaw and lower jaw, among which upper and lower jaw nerve pain are the most common. In most cases trigeminal neuralgia in both cheeks at the same time is seldom found.

Since such pain is short term and spasmodic, classic tranquilizers are usually ineffective. However acupoint stimulation using TCM techniques can produce good results.

Symptoms

Sharp pain suddenly attacks in the area of the trigeminal nerve in one side of face, just like an electric shock, cut, burn or prick. Some people tear up and run at the nose when it attacks.

Due to the sharp pain, the patient undertaking self-massage may often rub and knead the affected part excessively, leading to bruising and thickening of the skin or even wearing away the eyebrows. During attacks some people constantly suck their lips and chew in order to reduce the pain.

Light irritation may bring pain that only lasts for several seconds or a couple of moments each time. A convulsive twist will be felt in one side of the face. When the pain ceases, the affected side of the face will appear white first and then red, with conjunctival congestion, tears, runny nose and salivation.

Target Acupoints

Head and neck: Yangbai (GB 14), Taiyang (EX-HN 5), Quanliao (SI 18), Jiache (ST 6), Dicang (ST 4), Xiaguan (ST 7), Yingxiang (LI 20), Daying (ST 5).
Arms: Waiguan (SJ 5), Hegu (LI 4).

Recommended Massage

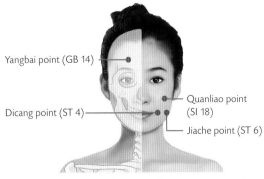

Yangbai point (GB 14)

Dicang point (ST 4)

Quanliao point (SI 18)

Jiache point (ST 6)

Location of the Yangbai, Quanliao, Jiache and Dicang points.

1. Pressing and Kneading the Yangbai Point
Location: Directly in line with the pupil, one cun above the eyebrow on the forehead.

Method: Lie on the back or sit upright. Use the index finger to gently press and knead the point for about two minutes, until some tingling and distension are felt as the best effect.

Effect: Cure facioplegia, drooping upper eyelids, supra-orbital neuralgia, facial convulsion, myopia, nyctalopia, acute conjunctivitis, nervous vomiting, headache, trigeminal pain and electric ophthalmia.

2. Pressing and Kneading the Quanliao Point

Location: Directly in the lower part of the outer canthus, in a cavity of the lower margin of the cheekbone.

Method: Lie on the back or sit upright. First use the index finger or thumb to press and knead the Quanliao point of the affected side for about 30 seconds. Then continue for another two minutes, until some tingling and distension are felt, ideally radiating all over the face.

Effect: Treat toothache, trifacial neuralgia, lower jaw arthritis, dislocation of lower jaw joints, convulsion of the masseter, facial convulsion, facioplegia, tympanitis, deafness and dumbness, dizziness and tinnitus.

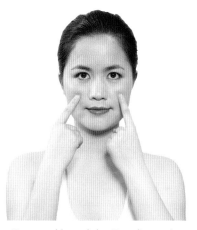

Press and knead the Quanliao point.

3. Pressing and Kneading the Jiache Point

Location: In a cavity about one cun in the upper part of the lower jaw corner, i.e. the highest point of the zygomaxillary muscle when one chews.

Method: Lie on the back or sit upright. Use the index finger to press and knead the Jiache point of the affected side for about two minutes, or press and knead it until the mouth secretes fluid.

Effect: Cure maxillary division or mandibular division pain of the trigeminal nerve, problems with the masseter, difficulty in opening the mouth, toothache, facioplegia, deviated mouth and eyes (facial paralysis), mouth watering, freckles and chloasma.

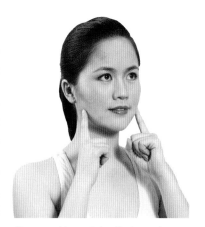

Press and knead the Jiache point.

4. Pressing and Kneading the Dicang Point

Location: About 0.4 cun away from the mouth corner, directly in line with the pupil.

Method: Lie on the back or sit upright. Use the index finger to gently press and knead the Dicang point of the affected side for two minutes with moderate force, until some tingling and distension are felt as the best effect.

Effect: Treat facioplegia, facial convulsion, trifacial neuralgia, mouth and lip edema, mouth and lip herpes, excessive salivation in children, angular stomatitis, toothache, gingivitis and oral ulcer.

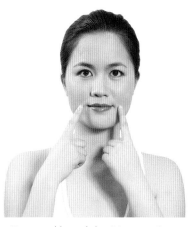

Press and knead the Dicang point.

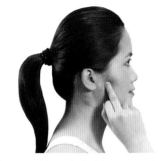

Press and knead the Xiaguan point.

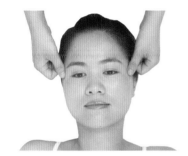

Press and knead the Taiyang point.

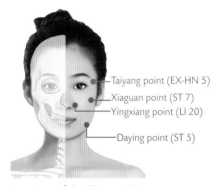

Taiyang point (EX-HN 5)
Xiaguan point (ST 7)
Yingxiang point (LI 20)

Daying point (ST 5)

Location of the Taiyang, Xiaguan, Yingxiang and Daying points.

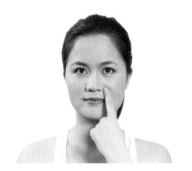

Press and knead the Yingxiang point.

5. Pressing and Kneading the Xiaguan Point

Location: In the depression at the hairline in front of the ear; it can be felt when the mouth is closed and creases when the mouth is open.

Method: Lie on the back or sit upright. Use the thumb tip to press and knead the Xiaguan point of the affected side for about 30 seconds and then continue for another two minutes, until some tingling and distension are felt, ideally radiating all over the face.

Effect: Treat toothache, trifacial neuralgia, difficulty in opening the mouth, deviated mouth and eyes (facial paralysis), and hyposiagonarthritis.

6. Pressing and Kneading the Taiyang Point

Location: In the depression about one cun behind the space between the outer tip of the brow and outer eye corner.

Method: Sit upright or lie on the back. Use the pad of the index finger to press the Taiyang points on both sides of the head, rubbing and kneading for two minutes until you feel tingling and expansion in the acupoints. If rubbing and kneading of a larger area is required, or you need more force, use the thenar eminences.

Effect: Cure cold, headache, fever, dizziness, and red and swollen eyes with pain.

7. Pressing and Kneading the Yingxiang Point

Location: Beside the wing of the nose, 0.5 cun away, in the nasolabial groove.

Method: Sitting upright, first use the index finger to press and knead the point for two minutes and then press for another 30 seconds, until some tingling and distension are felt as the best effect.

Effect: Excellent for easing various symptoms involving the nose, such as runny nose, nasal congestion, nose bleeding, nasosinusitis, decline of sense of smell, and chronic rhinitis. In addition this acupoint is also frequently used in cases of trifacial neuralgia and to treat the aftereffect of facial paralysis, as well as for facial beauty.

8. Pressing and Kneading the Daying Point

Location: In a cavity between the lip and lower jaw bone over the pulse of the facial artery.

Method: Use the index or middle finger to press the Daying point on both sides for about two minutes until some tingling and distension are felt, ideally radiating to the lower jaw and the neck.

Effect: Promote facial blood circulation and tighten the skin. It can eliminate double chin, prevent the facial skin from loosening, and cure toothache and oral ulcer.

9. Pressing and Kneading the Waiguan and Neiguan Points

Location: The Waiguan point is in the middle on the outside of the arm, between the ulna and radius about two cun away from the horizontal line of the wrist joint. The Neiguan point is between the two tendons about two cun above the wrist joint bend.

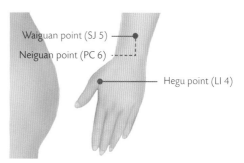

Location of the Hegu, Waiguan and Neiguan points.

Method: With the forearm bent halfway, use the thumb tip of one hand to press the Waiguan point in the other forearm, while using the index or middle finger to press the Neiguan point. Press them simultaneously 20 to 30 times, until tingling and distension are felt as the best effect.

Effect: Treat fever, cold, pneumonia, tinnitus, deafness, stiff neck, migraine, intercostal nerve pain, upper arm joint pain and elbow pain.

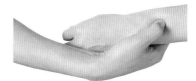

Press and knead the Waiguan and Neiguan points.

10. Pinching and Kneading the Hegu Point

Location: In the highest point on the back of the hand between the thumb base and the base of the index finger (in the webbing between these two fingers).

Method: Use the thumb tip of one hand to pinch the Hegu point on the other hand for about one minute, and continue pinching and kneading for about two minutes, until some tingling and distension are felt as the best effect.

Effect: Treat facioplegia, trigeminal pain, facial paralysis, deviated mouth and eyes (facial paralysis), rhinitis, headache, toothache, acne, visual fatigue, sore throat, tinnitus and hiccups.

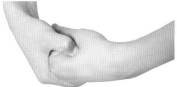

Press and knead the Hegu point.

Tips

Light trigeminal neuralgia in the early stage, or untypical trigeminal neuralgia, is often mistaken for toothache, migraine or ENT diseases. Some patients even have their teeth pulled without correct diagnosis, delaying timely treatment.

5 | Stiff Neck

Commonly there are no symptoms before one goes to bed. However one feels obvious tingling and pain in the neck and back in the morning, with neck movement restricted. It often takes place among young people, mostly in winter and spring.

Symptoms

It is mostly marked by pain, stiffness and restriction over neck movement and activities. Sometimes it is accompanied by pain in the upper corner of the scapula. Serious cases are marked by radiation of the pain to the head and back, even affecting arm movement. It takes a few days for recovery from a mild case but several weeks for a serious case.

Stiff neck is mostly caused by incorrect sleeping posture, cold infiltration into the muscles after hard work, sprain of the neck muscles and over stretching of the neck over a long time. It may develop into cervical spondylosis if it attacks frequently.

Target Acupoints

Head and neck: Pain point, Fengchi (GB 20).
Shoulder, back and waist: Tianzong (SI 11), Jianjing (GB 21), Feishu (BL 13).
Arms: Houxi (SI 3), Laozhen.
Legs: Chengjin (BL 56).

Recommended Massage

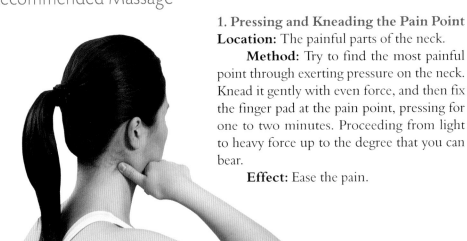

1. Pressing and Kneading the Pain Point
Location: The painful parts of the neck.

Method: Try to find the most painful point through exerting pressure on the neck. Knead it gently with even force, and then fix the finger pad at the pain point, pressing for one to two minutes. Proceeding from light to heavy force up to the degree that you can bear.

Effect: Ease the pain.

Press and knead the pain point.

2. Pressing and Kneading the Fengchi Point

Location: In the depression on both sides of the large tendon behind the nape of the neck, next to the lower edge of the skull.

Method: Sit upright. Use the pads of the thumbs or middle fingers to press the Fengchi point on both sides, proceeding from light to heavy force. Then knead gently until some tingling and distension are felt as the best effect. In the process of massage turn the neck gently. The massage generally lasts for two minutes or so.

Effect: Treat cold, fever, neck pain, headache, dizziness, and red and swollen eyes with pain.

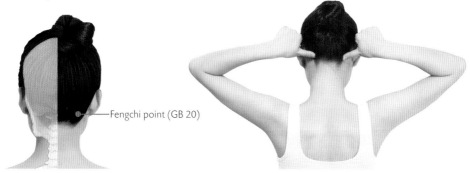

Fengchi point (GB 20)

Press and knead the Fengchi point.

3. Pressing and Kneading the Tianzong Point

Location: In the depression at the center of the scapula.

Method: Sit upright and relax the neck muscles. Use the middle finger to forcefully press and knead the Tianzong point of the affected side for two minutes. Ideally you should feel tingling and distension in the shoulder and back as well as weakness of the upper limbs. While massaging turn the neck slowly, proceeding from small to large scale movement.

Effect: Cure scapula pain, and trauma in the shoulder and back, as well as asthma.

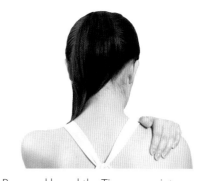

Press and knead the Tianzong point.

4. Kneading the Jianjing Point

Location: At the midpoint of the top on the shoulder.

Method: Sit upright. Use both middle fingers to press and knead the Jianjing point on both sides, with the palm heels and thenar eminences holding the upper part of the collarbone closely. The muscle in this area is lifted and pinched by the palms and

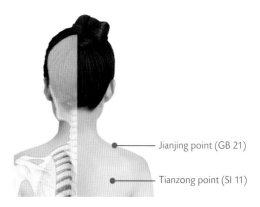

Jianjing point (GB 21)

Tianzong point (SI 11)

Location of the Jianjing, Feishu and Tianzong points.

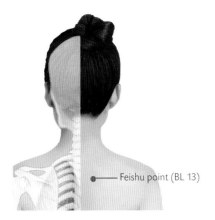

Feishu point (BL 13)

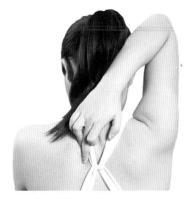

Press the Feishu point.

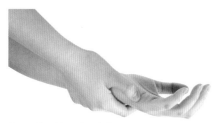

Press the Houxi point.

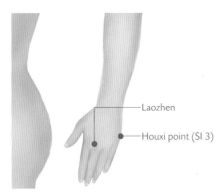

Laozhen

Houxi point (SI 3)

Location of the Laozhen and Houxi points.

fingers (with more force from the middle finger). Proceeding from light to heavy force, press, rub and knead the Jianjing point at the same time. Generally it takes two or three minutes until you feel relaxed in the shoulders and neck.

Effect: Treat cervical spondylosis, stiff neck, shoulder periarthritis, shoulder pain, inability to raise the arms, shoulder-back tingling and pain, sequela of apoplexy, difficult labor, fever and headache.

5. Pressing the Feishu Point

Location: At the point 1.5 cun beside the third thoracic vertebra on the inner side of the scapula.

Method: Sit on a chair. Use the middle finger to press the Feishu point of the opposite side. Use the palm of the other hand to raise the elbow of the opposite side. While pressing the Fengchi point, turn your body toward the other side of the Fengchi point.

Effect: Treat all kinds of diseases in the respiratory system (such as hematemesis, fever, difficulty in breathing), acne, fatigue all over the body, shoulder-back tingling and pain, dry skin, skin itch, spontaneous perspiration and night sweating.

6. Pressing the Houxi Point

Location: With the fist clenched, it is on the side of the hand, beside the last (largest) knuckle of the small finger.

Method: Use the thumbnail to press the Houxi point, proceeding from light to heavy force until tingling, numbness, heaviness and distension are felt upward.

Effect: Treat epilepsy, fever, malaria, deafness, red and swollen eyes, arm pain, chest pain, pain of cervical spondylosis and stiff neck.

7. Pressing the Laozhen Point

Location: At the point 0.5 cun between the second and third metacarpal bone behind the metacarpophalangeal joint.

Method: If the neck stiffness is on the left side, use the thumb of the right hand to press the Laozhen point on the left side for two minutes. Move the neck during the massage. Proceed from light to heavy force until tingling and distension are felt upward, ideally radiating directly to the neck. As for stiffness on the right side, use the thumb of the left hand.

Effect: Cure stiff neck and severe neck pain as well as pain, numbness, contracture or paralysis of the arms, and stomachalgia.

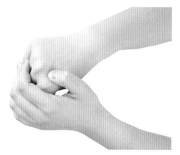

Press the Laozhen point.

8. Pressing and Kneading the Chengjin Point
Location: In the middle of the gastrocnemiu muscle; or on the highest prominence of the ca muscle if lying down or sitting upright with th foot slack.

Method: Sitting cross-legged, hold up on knee, fixed by one hand, while using the fu surface of the thumb of the other hand to pres and knead the Chengjin point in a circular manne You can also use the thumb to press and knead the Chengjin point of the affected side clockwise for two minutes, proceeding from light to heavy force, until tingling and distension are felt as the best effect.

Effect: Chiefly serves to cure waist and leg spasm, pain and hemorrhoids.

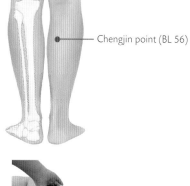

Chengjin point (BL 56)

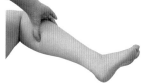

Press and knead the Chengjin point.

Tips
- Choose a proper pillow:
  - △ There should be a concave part in the middle to support the neck.
  - △ A pillow 8 to 10 centimeters high is suitable for women, and 10 to 15 centimeters high is suitable for men.
  - △ The pillow should not be too wide; the width is suitable if it is between the shoulder and the ear.
  - △ Correct softness is indicated by easy deformation.
- Be sure to keep warm. Cover the whole body and neck with a blanket. In hot weather do not expose the neck to an electric fan for a long time.
- People working at a desk for a long time should often raise the head and move it around in order to prevent chronic neck muscle strain.

6 Cervical Spondylosis

Also called cervical syndrome, it is a general term for osteoarthritis of the cervical spine, hyperplasia of cervical spondylosis, cervical nerve root syndrome and cervical disc herniation, as a type of disease based on degenerative changes.

Symptoms

Cervical spondylosis is marked by tingling and pain in the head, neck, shoulder, back and arm, as well as a stiff neck and restricted movement during activities.

The neck and shoulder pain can radiate to the head and arms, possibly coupled by dizziness and even in extreme cases by vomiting. A few patients may collapse.

When sympathetic nerves are affected by cervical spondylosis, there can be such symptoms as dizziness, headache, blurred eyesight, eye swelling, dry eyes, inability to open the eyes, tinnitus, loss of balance, tachycardia, palpitation, tightening in the chest, and even gastric and intestinal distension, generally accompanied by insomnia, agitation and depression.

Target Acupoints

Head and neck: Fengchi (GB 20), Tianyou (SJ 16).
Shoulder, back and waist: Jianjing (GB 21), Tianzong (SI 11).
Arms: Jianzhen (SI 9), Jiquan (HT 1), Waiguan (SJ 5), Hegu (LI 4).

Recommended Massage

1. Pressing and Kneading the Fengchi Point

Location: In the depression on both sides of the large tendon behind the nape of the neck, next to the lower edge of the skull.

Method: Sit upright, Place the pad of the thumb or the middle finger on the Fengchi point on both sides, pressing and kneading, proceeding from light to heavy force. During massage move the neck around gently. Knead lightly until you feel tingling and distension in the part concerned. The duration is generally about two minutes.

Effect: Cure cold, fever, neck pain, headache, dizziness, and red and swollen eyes with pain.

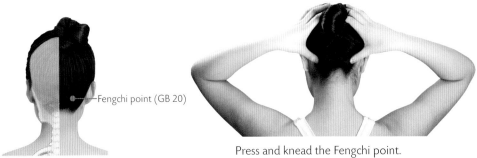

Fengchi point (GB 20)

Press and knead the Fengchi point.

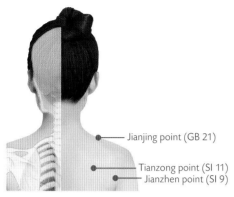

Jianjing point (GB 21)

Tianzong point (SI 11)
Jianzhen point (SI 9)

Location of the Fengchi, Jianjing, Tianzong and Jianzhen points.

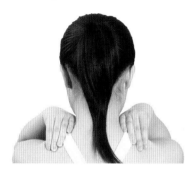

Knead the Jianjing point.

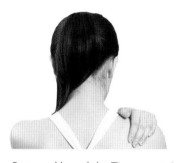

Press and knead the Tianzong point.

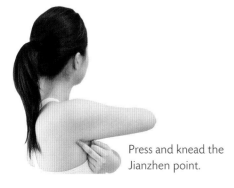

Press and knead the Jianzhen point.

2. Kneading the Jianjing Point

Location: At the midpoint of the top on the shoulder.

Method: Sit upright. Use both middle fingers to press and knead the Jianjing point on both sides, with the palm heels and thenar eminences holding the upper part of the collarbone closely. The muscle in this area is lifted and pinched by the palms and fingers (with more force from the middle finger). Proceeding from light to heavy force, press, rub and knead the Jianjing point at the same time. Generally it takes two or three minutes until you feel relaxed in the shoulders and neck. You can also do one side first and then the other side.

Effect: Treat cervical spondylosis, stiff neck, shoulder periarthritis, shoulder pain, inability to raise the arms, shoulder-back tingling and pain, sequela of apoplexy, difficult labor, fever and headache.

3. Pressing and Kneading the Tianzong Point

Location: In the depression at the center of the scapula.

Method: Sit upright. Relax the neck muscles and then use the middle finger to press, rub and knead the Tianzong point forcefully until you feel tingling and distension in the shoulder, and back and weakness in the arms.

Effect: Cure scapula pain, and trauma in the shoulder and back, as well as asthma.

4. Pressing and Kneading the Jianzhen Point

Location: At the lower back of the shoulder joint.

Method: Use the middle finger to press, rub and knead the Jianzhen point for two minutes with moderate force until you feel obviously tingling and distension in the part concerned.

Effect: Cure problems with the

shoulder joints and soft tissues around it as well as upper limb paralysis and armpit sweating.

5. Pressing and Kneading the Tianyou Point

Location: At the lower part of the mastoid process in a notch in the rear of the sternocleidomastoid, toward the back of the neck. This acupoint lies in the horizontal protruding part of the third cervical vertebra, which is where neck tingling and pain often attack since this part is quite long.

Method: Sit upright. Use the thumb pad surface to press, rub and knead for three minutes on both sides at the same time. Moderate force is applied until obvious tingling and distension are felt.

Effect: Cure headache, dizziness, stiff neck, sudden deafness and sore throat, in addition to scrofula and shoulder-back pain.

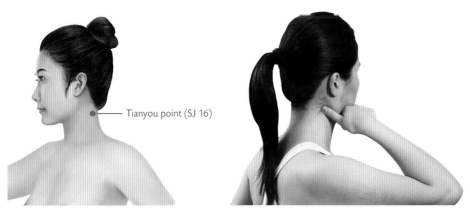

Press and knead the Tianyou point.

6. Pressing and Kneading the Jiquan Point

Location: In the middle of the armpit when the arm is raised.

Method: Sit upright with the arm raised. Use the middle finger pad of either hand to press the Jiquan point for two minutes forcefully until you feel tingling and distension, ideally radiating to the end of the fingers.

Effect: Cure numb and painful upper limbs, angina and bromhidrosis (body odor).

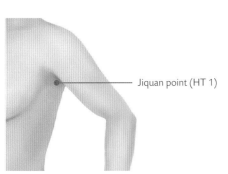

Press and knead the Jiquan point.

7. Pinching and Kneading the Hegu Point

Location: In the highest point on the back of the hand between the thumb base and the base of the index finger (in the webbing between these two fingers).

Method: Use the thumb to press the Hegu point on the other hand 10 to 20 times alternatively from light to heavy force until tingling and distension are felt as the best effect.

Effect: Cure cold, runny nose, headache, toothache, acne, visual fatigue, sore throat, tinnitus and hiccups.

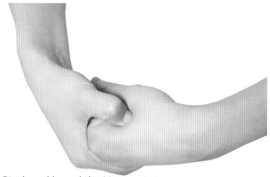

Pinch and knead the Hegu point.

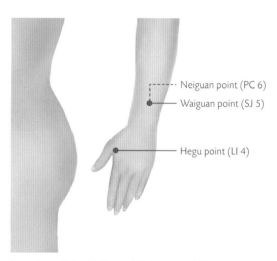

Neiguan point (PC 6)
Waiguan point (SJ 5)

Hegu point (LI 4)

Location of the Neiguan, Waiguan and Hegu points.

8. Pressing the Waiguan and Neiguan Points

Location: The Waiguan point is in the middle on the outside of the arm, between the ulna and radius about two cun away from the horizontal line of the wrist joint. The Neiguan point is between the two tendons about two cun above the wrist joint bend.

Method: With the arm bent halfway, use the thumb tip of the other hand to press the Waiguan point. At the same time use the index or middle finger to press the Neiguan point. In other words, both the Waiguan point and Neiquan point are pressed at the same time until tingling and distension are felt.

Effect: Treat fever, cold, pneumonia, tinnitus, deafness, stiff neck, migraine, intercostal nerve pain, and arm joint pain.

Tips

Patients with cervical spondylosis should:
- Pay attention to the position in which they work and study.
- Move the neck around moderately after working at a desk for a long time.
- Choose a pillow of appropriate height in order to prevent neck-oriented issues.

7 | Myopia

Myopia, which results in blurred eyesight when people look at things in the distance, is caused by hereditary factors, lights, sitting posture and improper use of the eyes. It happens mostly among young people and teenagers.

Clinically myopia involves convulsion of the ciliaris. In other words, gradually, the object in the distance cannot be concentrated in the retina itself but is focused at a point before it, leading to distorted eyesight and abnormal vision. It is pseudomyopia in the early stage. However it is apt to develop into true myopia over time.

If the adjustment of the ciliaris is imbalanced for a long time, there will be such symptoms as visual fatigue, nausea, swollen eyeballs with pain and even heterotropia.

Symptoms

The object in the distance looks blurred and unrecognizable, and patients may tend to squint. An imbalance between visual adjustment and concentration is caused since objects cannot be seen clearly. Vitreous opacity leads to flickering black shadows in the front when the eyeballs move around, mostly happening to people with myopia of intermediate degree or above. The eyeballs of people with myopia of high degree look slightly protruding since the optic axis is too long.

Target Acupoints

Head and neck: Jingming (BL 1), Sibai (ST 2), Yuyao (EX-HN 4), Taiyang (EX-HN 5), Fengchi (GB 20), Cuanzhu (BL 2), Sizhukong (SJ 23).
Arms: Shaoze (SI 1), Quchi (LI 11).
Legs: Guangming (GB 37).

Recommended Massage

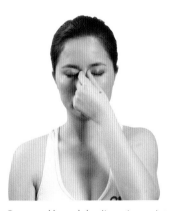

Press and knead the Jingming point.

1. **Pressing and Kneading the Jingming Point**
Location: In the depression over the inner corner of the eye.

Method: Lie on the back or sit upright. Use the tip of the thumb and the index or middle finger to press the Jingming points on both sides. With the onset of tingling and distension, proceed from light to heavy force, continuing for about two minutes until tingling and distension radiate to the eyes.

Effect: Ease visual fatigue, restore eyesight, and treat bloody eyes, red swelling, edema, glaucoma and cataract. In addition it can ease nasal congestion if acupoints around the nose are massaged at the same time.

2. Pressing and Kneading the Sibai Point

Location: Directly below the pupil, in a cavity below the orbit.

Method: Use the pads of the middle fingers to press the Sibai point on both sides. When there is tingling and pain, gradually increase force, pressing and kneading for about two minutes, so that the radiating tingling and distension reaches to the eyes.

Effect: It has a very good effect on symptoms caused by facioplegia such as failure to open and close the eyes, pain near the cheeks, trigeminal pain, myopia, visual fatigue and giddiness.

3. Pressing and Kneading the Yuyao Point

Location: Directly above the pupil in the middle of each eyebrow.

Method: Use the pads of the two index or middle fingers to gently press and knead the Yuyao points above the eyes for two minutes, until tingling and distension are felt as the best effect.

Effect: Cure forehead pain, drooping eyelids, red and swollen eyes with pain, slight corneal opacity and myopia.

4. Pressing and Kneading the Taiyang Point

Location: In the depression about one cun behind the space between the outer tip of the brow and outer eye corner.

Method: Use the pads of both index fingers to press the Taiyang points on both sides for about two minutes until some tingling and distension are felt as the best effect. If a larger area or heavier force is required, you can use both thenar eminences to knead them gently, concentrating at the Taiyang point.

Effect: Cure cold, headache, fever, dizziness, and red and swollen eyes with pain.

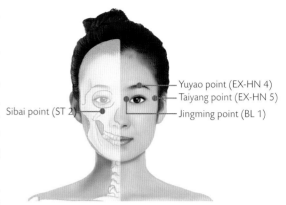

Sibai point (ST 2) — Yuyao point (EX-HN 4) — Taiyang point (EX-HN 5) — Jingming point (BL 1)

Location of the Yuyao, Jingming, Taiyang and Sibai points.

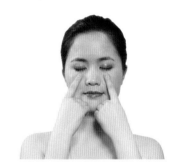

Press and knead the Sibai point.

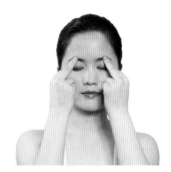

Press and knead the Yuyao point.

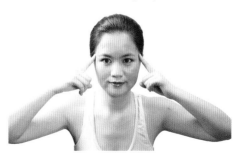

Press and knead the Taiyang point.

5. Pressing and Kneading the Cuanzhu Point

Location: In a cavity where the inner eyebrow starts.

Method: Use the pad of the index finger to press the Cuanzhu point of the affected side. When there are tingling and distension, proceed from light to heavy force for about two minutes until tingling and distension radiate to the eyes.

Effect: It has a very good effect on eye tearing, dizziness, visual fatigue, eye edema, conjunctivitis, cheek pain, headache and high blood pressure. The Cuanzhu point is also often used in facial beauty treatment.

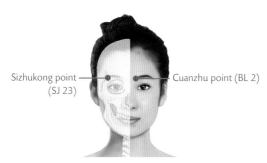

Sizhukong point (SJ 23)

Cuanzhu point (BL 2)

Location of the Sizhukong and Cuanzhu points.

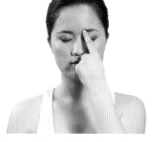

Press and knead the Cuanzhu point.

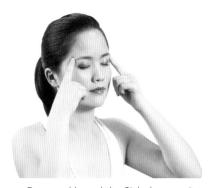

Press and knead the Sizhukong point.

6. Pressing and Kneading the Sizhukong Point

Location: In a cavity near the outer eyebrow tip.

Method: Use the pad of the index finger to press the Sizhukong point. When there are tingling and distension, proceed from light to heavy force for about two minutes, ideally until the effect radiates to the eyes.

Effect: It is often used in eye beauty therapy, serving to prevent lines and dark circles, in addition to curing headache, swollen and painful eyes, twitching eyelids and toothache.

7. Pressing and Kneading the Fengchi Point

Location: In the depression on both sides of the large tendon behind the nape of the neck, next to the lower edge of the skull.

Method: Sit upright. Use the pads of both thumbs to press the Fengchi point on both sides while using the rest of the fingers to hold the head. Press and knead for two minutes, proceeding from light to heavy force, continuing to press for another 30 seconds until some tingling and distension are felt as the best effect. Ideally distension and numbness will progress to the temples.

Effect: Treat cold, fever, neck pain, headache, dizziness, and red and swollen eyes with pain.

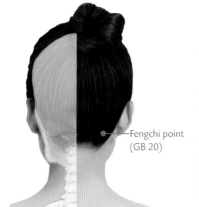

Fengchi point (GB 20)

Location of the Fengchi point.

8. Pressing the Shaoze Point

Location: At the bottom corner of the nail bed on the outer side of the small finger.

Method: Use the thumb and index finger to hold the end of the small finger of the other hand while using the thumb tip to press the Shaoze point.

Effect: Prevent the decline of eyesight.

9. Pressing and Kneading the Quchi Point

Location: With the elbow bent halfway, on the outer side of the cubital transverse crease.

Method: Use the thumb to press and knead the Quchi point in the other arm in a small circle. Use force from the elbow to help exert pressure with the finger.

Effect: Maintain normal visual nerve functions.

10. Pinching and Kneading the Guangming Point

Location: On the front edge of the fibula, 5 cun over the lateral malleolus.

Method: Lie on a chair and stretch the legs. Use two thumbs to pinch and knead the Guangming point of both sides, first for two minutes. Then continue to press another 30 seconds until tingling and distension become obvious.

Effect: Treat various eye issues, such as visual fatigue, red swelling, trachoma, bloodshot eyes, decline of eyesight, blurred eyesight and amblyopia (lazy eye).

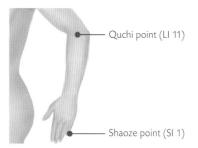

Quchi point (LI 11)

Shaoze point (SI 1)

Location of the Quchi and Shaoze points.

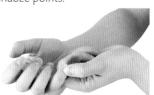

Press the Shaoze point.

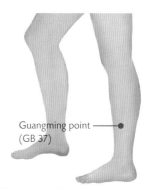

Guangming point (GB 37)

Location of the Guangming point.

Tips

Despite the many advantages of contact lenses, attention should be paid to the following recommendations:

- Do not wear contact lenses for a period of more than 72 hours, in order to reduce eye complications and prolong the lifespan of the contact lenses.
- Be sure to sterilize the contact lenses, putting them in and taking them out only after cleaning the hands.
- Do not wear contact lenses in a polluted environment.
- Pay close attention to the eye's reaction after putting on contact lenses, taking them off immediately when something unusual occurs, and seeking medical attention for severe reactions.
- It is best to have a pair of ordinary glasses as a back-up.

8 Optic Nerve Atrophy

This refers to the degenerative change of the optic nerve fibers, which impairs visual functions.

The reasons for this illness are quite complex. Generally speaking in children it is mostly caused by brain tumors or intracranial inflammation. Young patients chiefly suffer from hereditary optic nerve atrophy. Middle-aged patients mostly suffer from optic neuritis, trauma of the optic nerve or oppression by tumors in the optic cross area within the brain. Optic nerve atrophy of old patients is often associated with glaucoma or vascular diseases.

Symptoms

It is chiefly marked by the decline of eyesight, contraction of the range of vision, dark spots at the center and difficulty in distinguishing colors. Severe cases can lead to blindness. The varied reasons for the illness can lead to different symptoms. Primary optic nerve atrophy is featured by a pale optic disc, and the blood vessels of the optic retina become fine while blood capillaries disappear. With secondary optic nerve atrophy the optic disc looks gray, wax yellow or light red, with disappearance of physiologic depression. In addition the blood vessels of the optic retina become fine.

Watching a screen for too long is apt to lead to optic nerve atrophy. One should seek medical attention as soon as possible if one fails to see clearly due to obvious decline of eyesight, or experiences a decrease in the range of vision, dilated pupils and sensitivity to light. You should also see a doctor if the eyes turn red with sensations of burning or hosting a foreign body, or you experience heavy eyelids, blurred eyesight and even swelling pain in the eyeball or headache that does not improve after rest.

Target Acupoints

Head and neck: Cuanzhu (BL 2), Jingming (BL 1), Qiuhou (EX-HN 7), Tongziliao (GB 1), Fengchi (GB 20), Yuyao (EX-HN 4), Chengqi (ST 1), Sibai (ST 2).
Legs: Guangming (GB 37).

Recommended Massage

1. Pressing and Kneading the Qiuhou Point
Location: Just below the eye, halfway between the pupil and the outer corner.

Method: Use the pad of the index finger to press the Qiuhou point of the affected side. When there are tingling and distension, proceed from light to heavy force, continuing for about two minutes until tingling and distension radiate to the eyes.

Effect: Treat optic neuritis, retinitis pigmentosa, vitreous opacity, glaucoma, early-stage cataract, myopia, heterotropia and fundus hemorrhage.

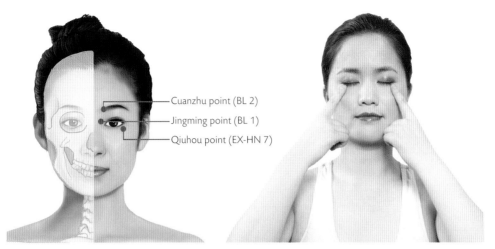

Location of the Cuanzhu, Jingming and Qiuhou points.

Press and knead the Qiuhou point.

2. Pressing and Kneading the Jingming Point

Location: In the depression over the inner corner of the eye.

Method: Lie on the back or sit upright. Use the thumb tip, index finger or middle finger to press the Jingming point of the affected side, pressing the inner upper part for two minutes until some tingling and distension are felt as the best effect.

Effect: Ease fatigue and restore eyesight, as well as treat bloodshot eyes, red swelling, edema, glaucoma and cataract. In addition it can ease nasal congestion when accompanied by massage of acupoints around the nose.

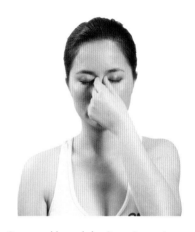

Press and knead the Jingming point.

3. Pressing and Kneading the Cuanzhu Point

Location: In a cavity where the inner eyebrow starts.

Method: Use the pad of the middle finger to press the Cuanzhu point on the affected side. When there is a sense of tingling and distension, gradually increase force until tingling and distension radiate to the eyes, pressing for about two minutes in total.

Effect: It has a very good effect on eye tearing, dizziness, visual fatigue, eye edema, conjunctivitis, cheek pain, headache and high blood pressure. The Cuanzhu point is also often used in facial beauty treatment.

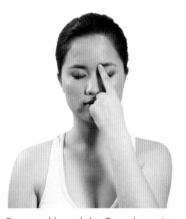

Press and knead the Cuanzhu point.

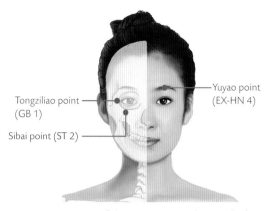

Location of the Yuyao, Tongziliao, and Sibai points.

Tongziliao point (GB 1)

Yuyao point (EX-HN 4)

Sibai point (ST 2)

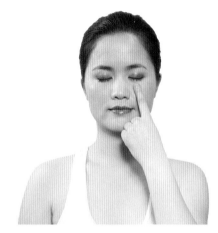

Press and knead the Sibai point.

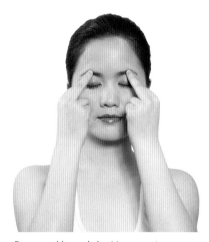

Press and knead the Yuyao point.

4. Pressing and Kneading the Sibai Point

Location: Directly below the pupil, in a cavity below the orbit.

Method: Use the pads of the index fingers to press the Sibai point on both sides. When there is tingling and pain, gradually increase force, pressing and kneading for about two minutes, so that the radiating tingling and distension reaches to the eyes.

Effect: It has a very good effect on symptoms caused by facioplegia such as failure to open and close the eyes, pain near the cheeks, trigeminal pain, myopia, visual fatigue and giddiness. In addition it is also an acupoint frequently used in facial beauty therapy.

5. Pressing and Kneading the Tongziliao Point

Location: At the point 0.5 cun laterally outside of the outer canthus.

Method: Use the pad of the index finger to press the Tongziliao point of the affected side. When there is tingling and pain, increase force to press and knead for two minutes, radiating the tingling and distension to the eyes.

Effect: It has a very good effect on curing headache, dizziness, seeing stars, visual fatigue, eye itch and conjunctival congestion. It is also an important acupoint for eye beauty therapy.

6. Pressing and Kneading the Yuyao Point

Location: Directly above the pupil in the middle of each eyebrow.

Method: Use the pads of the two index or middle fingers to gently press and knead the Yuyao points above the eyes for two minutes, until tingling and distension are felt as the best effect.

Effect: Cure forehead pain, drooping eyelids, red and swollen eyes with pain, slight corneal opacity and myopia.

7. Pressing and Kneading the Chengqi Point

Location: Directly below the pupil, between the lower edge of the eyeball and the eye socket.

Method: Use the tip of the index finger to press the Chengqi point of the affected side along the infraorbital margin. Press the eyeball carefully using only moderate force until tingling and distension are obvious.

Effect: Prevent tears caused by wind, myopia, nyctalopia, twitching eyelids, deviated mouth and eyes (facial paralysis) and facial convulsion.

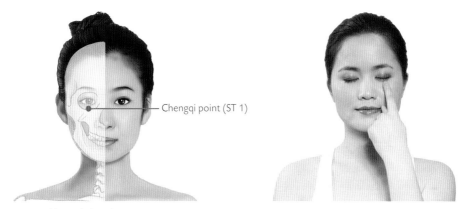

Chengqi point (ST 1)

Press and knead the Chengqi point.

8. Pressing and Kneading the Fengchi Point

Location: In the depression on both sides of the large tendon behind the nape of the neck, next to the lower edge of the skull.

Method: Sit upright. Use the pads of both thumbs to press the Fengchi point of both sides for 30 seconds at first, then continue to press and knead for another two minutes. Move from light to heavy force until you feel obvious tingling and distension as the best effect.

Effect: Treat cold, fever, neck pain, headache, dizziness, and red and swollen eyes with pain.

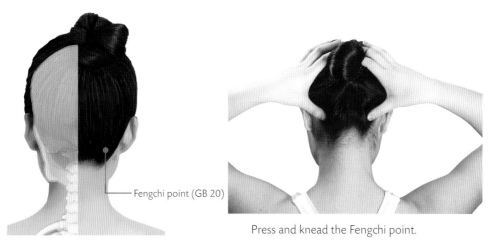

Fengchi point (GB 20)

Press and knead the Fengchi point.

9. Pressing and Pinching the Guangming Point

Location: On the front edge of the fibula, 5 cun over the lateral malleolus.

Method: Lie on a chair and stretch the legs. Use two thumbs to press and pinch the Guangming point of both sides for two minutes. Then continue to press for another 30 seconds until tingling and distension are obviously felt.

Effect: Treat various eye diseases, such as visual fatigue, red swelling, trachoma, bloodshot eyes, blurred eyesight and amblyopia.

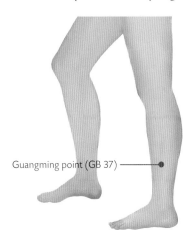

Guangming point (GB 37)

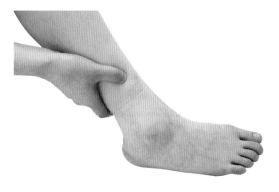

Press and pinch the Guangming point.

Tips

- Avoid direct strong light.
- Do not stay in an environment where the air conditioning runs continually; avoid air flow blowing across one's self.
- Use a humidifier or boiling water nearby to increase humidity in the nearby environment.
- Do not stare for long periods of time. Blinking the eyes frequently can prevent them from being exposed to the air for a long time, avoiding evaporation of tears.
- Frequent computer users should pay attention to the following points:
  - △ Those above the age of 40 should consider using bifocal or lower-degree glasses when at the computer.
  - △ Adjust the distance between oneself and the screen, with a distance of 50 to 70 centimeters suggested. The screen should be 10 to 20 centimeters lower than eye level, providing a downward optic angle of 15 to 20 degrees.
  - △ Keep a correct work posture. Look horizontally or look slightly down at the screen so as to relax the neck muscles.
  - △ Take a five to ten minutes rest for every hour of continuous work. During the rest period, look into the distance or do eye exercises.

9 Acute Conjunctivitis

It is chiefly marked by acute conjunctival congestion and the increase of secretion. This may be coupled with light sensitivity, tears, pain and itchiness, or burning and sticky tears. The eyelids of children will be more swollen and reddish than those of adult patients.

Symptoms

There are two types of conjunctivitis, bacterial and viral.

With bacterial conjunctivitis, there is obvious conjunctival congestion along with pus or oozing secretion, the sensation of a foreign body lodged in the eye, burning, prickling pain, and slight light sensitivity. The patient will still have sound eyesight. The secretion may be of bloody color. A gray membrane can be seen on the eyelid conjunctiva. Such membrane can be removed by a cotton swab but will reoccur easily.

In cases of viral conjunctivitis, there will be red eyes with edema and possible bleeding, accompanied by watery or sticky secretion, tear shedding and the sensation of a foreign body. The eyesight can be affected due to small fine and white turbid spots in the cornea, or it may lead to lymphadenectasis of the same side, with the area before the ear exhibiting pain if pressed.

Target Acupoints

Head and neck: Jingming (BL 1), Chengqi (ST 1), Sibai (ST 2), Taiyang (EX-HN 5), Cuanzhu (BL 2), Yuyao (EX-HN 4) and Fengchi (GB 20).
Arms: Hegu (LI 4), Waiguan (SJ 5).
Legs: Yanglingquan (GB 34).

Recommended Massage

1. Pressing and Kneading the Jingming Point
Location: In the depression over the inner corner of the eye.

Method: Lie on the back or sit upright. Use the thumb tip, index finger or middle finger to press the Jingming point of the affected side, pressing the inner upper part for two minutes until some tingling and distension are felt as the best effect.

Effect: Ease fatigue and restore

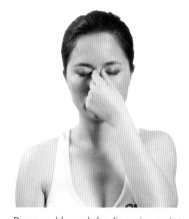

Press and knead the Jingming point.

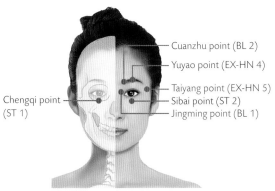

Cuanzhu point (BL 2)

Yuyao point (EX-HN 4)

Taiyang point (EX-HN 5)

Chengqi point (ST 1)

Sibai point (ST 2)

Jingming point (BL 1)

Location of the Cuanzhu, Yuyao, Jingming, Taiyang, Chengqi and Sibai points.

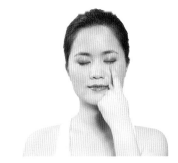

Press and knead the Chengqi point.

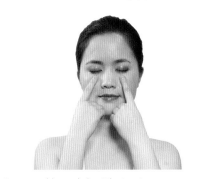

Press and knead the Sibai point.

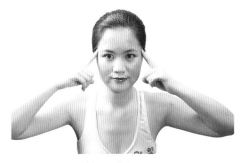

Press and knead the Taiyang point.

eyesight, as well as treat bloodshot eyes, red swelling, edema, glaucoma and cataract. In addition it can ease nasal congestion when accompanied by massage of acupoints around the nose.

2. Pressing and Kneading the Chengqi Point

Location: Directly below the pupil, between the lower edge of the eyeball and the eye socket.

Method: Use the tip of the index finger to press the Chengqi point of the affected side along the infraorbital margin. Press the eyeball carefully using only moderate force until tingling and distension are obvious.

Effect: Prevent tears caused by wind, myopia, nyctalopia, twitching eyelids, deviated mouth and eyes (facial paralysis) and facial convulsion.

3. Pressing and Kneading the Sibai Point

Location: Directly below the pupil, in a cavity below the orbit.

Method: Use the pads of the index fingers to press the Sibai point on both sides. When there is tingling and pain, gradually increase force, pressing and kneading for about two minutes, so that the radiating tingling and distension reaches to the eyes.

Effect: It has a very good effect on symptoms caused by facioplegia such as failure to open and close the eyes, pain near the cheeks, trigeminal pain, myopia, visual fatigue and giddiness. In addition it is also an acupoint frequently used in facial beauty therapy.

4. Pressing and Kneading the Taiyang Point

Location: In the depression about one cun behind the space between the outer tip of the brow and outer eye corner.

Method: Sit upright or lie on the back. Use the pad of the index finger to press the Taiyang points on both sides of the head, rubbing and kneading for two minutes until you feel tingling and expansion in the acupoints. If rubbing and kneading of a larger area is required, or you need more force, use the thenar eminences.

Effect: Cure cold, headache, fever, dizziness, and red and swollen eyes with pain.

5. Pressing and Kneading the Cuanzhu Point

Location: In a cavity where the inner eyebrow starts.

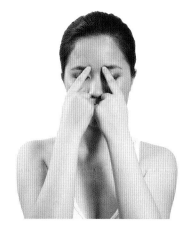

Method: Use the pad of the index finger to press and knead the Cuanzhu point on the affected side. When there is a sense of tingling and distension, gradually increase force until tingling and distension radiate to the eyes, pressing for about two minutes in total.

Effect: It has a very good effect on eye tearing, dizziness, visual fatigue, eye edema, conjunctivitis, cheek pain, headache and high blood pressure. The Cuanzhu point is also often used in facial beauty treatment.

Press and knead the Cuanzhu point.

6. Pressing and Kneading the Yuyao Point

Location: Directly above the pupil in the middle of each eyebrow.

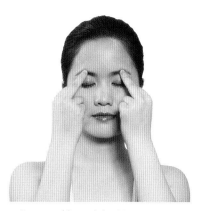

Method: Use the pads of the two index or middle fingers to gently press and knead the Yuyao points above the eyes for two minutes, until some tingling and distension are felt as the best effect.

Effect: Cure forehead pain, drooping eyelids, red and swollen eyes with pain, slight corneal opacity and myopia.

Press and knead the Yuyao point.

7. Pressing and Kneading the Fengchi Point

Location: In the depression on both sides of the large tendon behind the nape of the neck, next to the lower edge of the skull.

Method: Sit upright. Place the pads of the middle and index fingers of both hands on the Fengchi point on either side of the head. Press and knead for two minutes proceeding from light to heavy force. Then press the Fengchi point for another 30 seconds, until you feel tingling and distension in the related part.

Effect: Treat cold, fever, neck pain, headache, dizziness, and red and swollen eyes with pain.

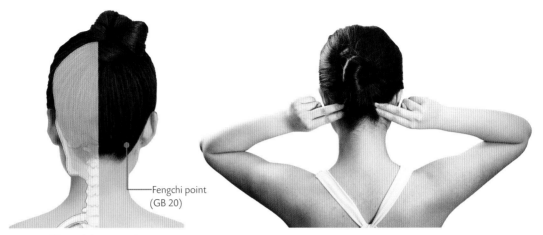

Fengchi point
(GB 20)

Press and knead the Fengchi point

8. Pressing the Waiguan and Neiguan Points

Location: The Waiguan point is in the middle on the outside of the arm, between the ulna and radius about two cun away from the horizontal line of the wrist joint. The Neiguan point is between the two tendons about two cun above the wrist joint bend.

Method: With the front arm bent halfway, use one thumb tip to press the Waiguan point on the other arm. The index or middle finger should press the Neiguan point, pressing inward 20 to 30 times, until tingling and distension are felt.

Effect: Cure fever, cold, pneumonia, tinnitus, dumbness, stiff neck, migraine, intercostal nerve pain, upper limb joint pain, and elbow pain.

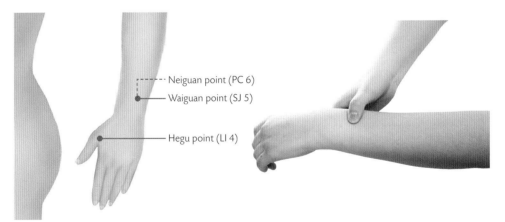

Neiguan point (PC 6)
Waiguan point (SJ 5)

Hegu point (LI 4)

Location of the Neiguan, Waiguan and Hegu point.   Press the Neiguan and Waiguan points.

9. Pinching and Kneading the Hegu Point

Location: In the highest point on the back of the hand between the thumb base and the base of the index finger (in the webbing between these two fingers).

Method: Lie on the back or sit upright. Use the thumb of one hand to press the Hegu point of the other hand, proceeding from light to heavy force. Press 10 to

20 times, with two hands used alternately, until tingling and distension are felt as the best effect.

Effect: Treat cold, runny nose, headache, toothache, acne, visual fatigue, sore throat, tinnitus and hiccups.

10. Pinching the Yanglingquan Point

Location: On the outer side of the shin in a notch at the front lower part of the fibula.

Method: Sit upright. Use the thumb tip to pinch the Yanglingquan point forcefully, with pressure directed toward the toes for about one minute, until obvious tingling and distension are felt as the best effect.

Effect: Cure migraine, dizziness, red face, red eyes, sore throat, toothache, acne, hives, erysipelas and arm pain.

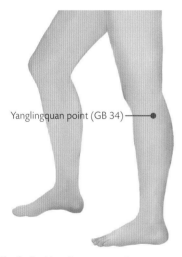
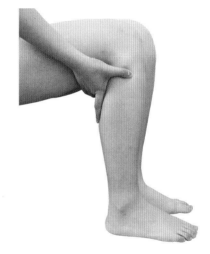

Yanglingquan point (GB 34)

Pinch the Yanglingquan point.

Tips
- To avoid cross-infection, when putting in eye drops, if only one eye is affected, lie on the side with the affected eye lower. This will prevent the healthy eye from being infected.
- Before and after applying eye drops, wash hands thoroughly. If someone is assisting in putting in the drops, they should also wash hands before and after.
- Do not rub the eyes in case of infection.
- Acute conjunctivitis is highly infectious. One's towel and other personal articles should be washed in hot water every day. Personal articles should not be shared in order to prevent infection.

10 | Tinnitus

This refers to hearing unusual sound, often ringing, that has no outside source. It is more obvious in a quiet environment.

This is a symptom resulting from a disorder of the hearing function. Clinically it may accompany many kinds of diseases, often in relation to high blood pressure, neurosis, drug poisoning and tympanic membrane defect caused by trauma (by sound or other impact). The disease is often regarded as a precursor of deafness.

Great strain, stress and exhaustion over a long time are apt to make tinnitus worse.

Symptoms

Tinnitus can be divided into two categories: continuous and rhythmic. With continuous tinnitus, it can be of a single frequency or a mixture of frequencies. In most cases of rhythmic tinnitus, it coincides with the pulse of blood vessels and occasionally with breathing. Tinnitus is usually marked by low frequency. However its frequency will be quite high if it is caused by muscular contraction.

Target Acupoints

Head and neck: Touqiaoyin (GB 11), Ermen (SJ 21), Tinggong (SI 19), Tinghui (GB 2), Yifeng (SJ 17), Shuaigu (GB 8), Tianzhu (BL 10), Fengchi (GB 20).
Shoulder, back and waist: Ganshu (BL 18), Shenshu (BL 23).

Recommended Massage

1. Pressing the Tinggong Point
Location: With the mouth open, in a cavity before the tragus on a line with the earlobe.

Method: Use the radialis of the thumbs to massage the Tinggong points on both sides, up and down 10 to 20 times. Then use the thumb tip to press the Tinggong point for one minute while opening the mouth slightly. There will be slight warmth during massage as well as an alternating feeling of blockage and openness inside the ears that accompanies the pressing. Upon completion there should be an improvement of hearing.

Effect: The Tinggong point is an acupoint with a special effect on curing tinnitus and hearing difficulty. Massaging this acupoint is also effective in curing headache, dizziness, decline of eyesight, and deterioration of memory linked to problems with ear and facial muscles (since the inner systems of the head are closely related and influence one another).

2. Pressing the Ermen Point

Location: With the mouth open, in a cavity before the notch of the tragus, behind the mandibular condyle.

Method: Use the radialis of the thumbs to massage the Ermen point on both sides, up and down 10 to 20 times. Then use the thumb tip to press the Ermen point for one minute while opening the mouth slightly. There will be slight warmth during massage as well as an alternating feeling of blockage and openness inside the ears that accompanies the pressing.

Effect: Treat tinnitus, deafness, toothache and neck-jaw pain.

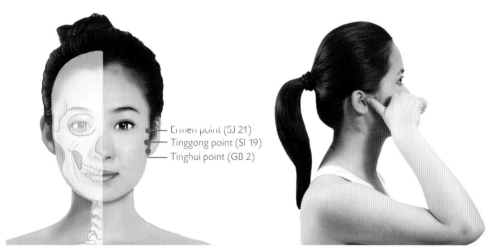

Location of the Ermen, Tinggong and Tinghui points.   Press the Tinggong point.

3. Pressing and Kneading the Tinghui Point

Location: With the mouth open, in a cavity before the intertragic notch behind the mandibular condyle.

Method: Use the radialis of the thumbs to massage the Tinghui point on both sides for two minutes, then use the thumb tip to press it for another 30 seconds. Open the mouth slightly when pressing, massaging until some tingling and distension are obviously felt.

Effect: Treat tinnitus, deafness, toothache and neck-jaw pain.

4. Pressing the Touqiaoyin Point

Location: In back of the ear, at about the halfway point of the ear approximately level with the helix root.

Method: Use two index fingers to press the Touqiaoyin point of both sides vertically 20 to 30 times until tingling and distension are felt as the best effect.

Effect: Treat head and neck pain, ear pain, tinnitus, deafness and sore throat.

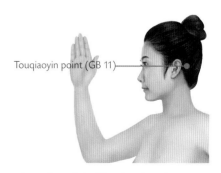

Location of the Touqiaoyin point.

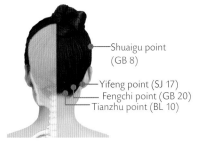

Shuaigu point
(GB 8)

Yifeng point (SJ 17)
Fengchi point (GB 20)
Tianzhu point (BL 10)

Location of the Shuaigu, Yifeng,
Fengchi amd Tianzhu points.

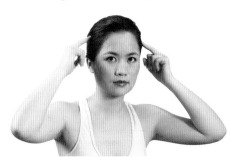

Press and knead the Shuaigu point.

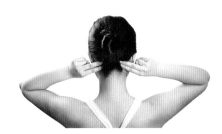

Press and knead the Fengchi point.

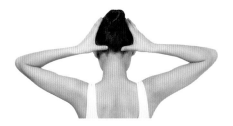

Press the Tianzhu point.

5. Pressing and Kneading the Shuaigu Point

Location: On the side of the head, four centimeters above the tip of the ear.

Method: Lie on the back or sit upright. First use the middle finger to press and knead the Shuaigu point for two minutes, then continue to press it for another 30 seconds until some tingling and distension are felt.

Effect: Often serve to cure vascular nervous headache, nervous tinnitus (deafness) and conjunctivitis.

6. Pressing and Kneading the Fengchi Point

Location: In the depression on both sides of the large tendon behind the nape of the neck, next to the lower edge of the skull.

Method: Sit upright. Use the pads of the middle and index fingers of both hands to press the Fengchi point on both sides, proceeding from light to heavy force. Generally one should press for 30 seconds and knead for two minutes until tingling and distension spreads to the ears.

Effect: Treat cold, fever, neck pain, headache, dizziness, and red and swollen eyes with pain.

7. Pressing the Tianzhu Point

Location: At the rear of the head, 1.5 cun from the middle line and one cun above the hairline.

Method: Using the thumb, press the Tianzhu point of the same side of the head. As the head turns to the other side, the thumb should press downwards on the Tianzhu point in a slanting manner.

Effect: Get rid of cold, tranquilize the spirit, and cure fever, dizziness, neck-shoulder tingling and pain, cervical spondylosis, drowsiness, fatigue, low blood pressure, high blood pressure, drunkenness and car sickness.

8. Pressing and Kneading the Yifeng Point

Location: Behind the earlobe in a notch between the mastoid process and the lower frontal angle.

Method: Place the tip of the index or middle finger on the Yifeng point, pressing and then rubbing and kneading, moving from light to heavy force. Usually pressing lasts for 30 seconds, followed by rubbing and kneading for two minutes until you feel tingling and distension at the Yifeng point. Ideally this feeling will radiate to the inner ears.

Effect: Cure deafness, tinnitus, dumbness, facioplegia, facial convulsion, trifacial neuralgia, tympanitis, external otitis (ear infection), tonsil inflammation, mandibular arthritis, stomatitis, hypertrophy of thyroid glands, toothache, eye disease, migraine and phrenospasm (spasm of the diaphragm).

9. Pressing the Ganshu Point

Location: 1.5 cun away from the ninth thoracic spinal process on the inner side of the scapula.

Method: Sit upright. Use the knuckles of the four fingers to knead the Ganshu point for about two minutes until tingling and distension are felt.

Effect: Treat distension and pain of both sides of the chest, breast pain with swelling, waist-back pain, agitation, irritability, indigestion and aversion to food, neurasthenia, hepatitis, jaundice (icterus), nausea, vomiting, lack of appetite and dizziness.

10. Pressing and Kneading the Shenshu Point

Location: 1.5 cun horizontally from the second lumbar spinal process.

Method: Lie on the back or sit upright. Use the two middle fingers to forcefully press and knead the Shenshu point of both sides 30 to 50 times, keeping the thumbs by the ribs. Or, with a clenched fist, use the knuckle of the index finger to press and knead the Shenshu point 30 to 50 times. You might also try using a loose fist to knead and rub 30 to 50 times, until some warmth is felt as the best effect.

Effect: Treat waist tingling and leg pain, lumbar muscle strain, lumbar disc herniation, leg swelling, fatigue all over the body, impotence, nocturnal emission, premature ejaculation and menstrual disorder.

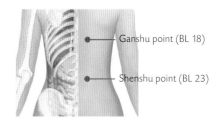

Ganshu point (BL 18)

Shenshu point (BL 23)

Location of the Ganshu and Shenshu points.

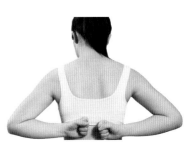

Press the Ganshu point.

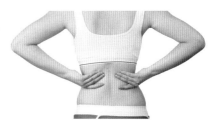

Press and knead the Shenshu point.

Tips

Those suffering from tinnitus should pay attention to the following in their daily life:

- Try to avoid loud noise and do not use earphones at a high volume.
- Relax the mind.
- Moderate your work rhythm.
- Engage in healthy and interesting hobbies and activities, but try to avoid doing complex, heavy and tiring things.

11 | Toothache

Toothache can be caused by any kind of problem with the teeth. Gingivitis, periodontitis, tooth decay and pulpitis are stomatological diseases that often lead to toothache.

In addition toothache can also be caused by neglect of oral hygiene, incorrect brushing of the teeth, vitamin deficiency, and long-term irritation from tartar and calculus formed by food residues and infection.

Some diseases of the nervous system can cause toothache such as trifacial neuralgia and peripheral facial neuritis. Chronic diseases can also result in toothache, as a complication of high blood pressure or diabetes for example.

Symptoms

With the so-called "hot wind-oriented" toothache, pain is periodic, attacking when the tooth is exposed to the wind. The pain of the affected part diminishes when it feels cold and increases when it feels hot. The pulp is swollen. The patient may have an overall feeling of fever, severe cold, thirst, and red tongue or white coating on a dry tongue.

When the toothache is related to gastric heat, as classified by TCM, the pain attacks sharply along with swollen pulp or the outbreak of pustules and bleeding. The swelling extends to the cheeks, leading to headache, thirst, bad breath, constipation, and yellow and thick coating on the tongue.

Toothache of deficiency-oriented heat is marked by faint or slight pain, along with slightly red pulp and minor swelling. Gradually there will be pulp contraction, loosened teeth, weakness of the teeth when biting into food, greater pain after noon, tingling and pain all over the body, dizziness, blurred vision, thirst without the desire to drink, and red and tender coating on the tongue.

Target Acupoints

Head and neck: Xiaguan (ST 7), Jiache (ST 6), Fengchi (GB 20), Pain point, Daying (ST 5).
Arms: Hegu (LI 4), Waiguan (SJ 5).
Legs: Taixi (KI 3).

Recommended Massage

1. Pressing and Kneading the Pain Point
Location: The most painful point of toothache.

Method: Use the pad of the index finger or the side of the thumb to press and knead the most painful point of toothache, proceeding from light to heavy force. Continue for about two minutes until tingling or distension are felt, leading to gradual alleviation of the pain.

Effect: Ease pain.

2. Pressing and Kneading the Xiaguan Point

Location: In the depression at the hairline in front of the ear; it can be felt when the mouth is closed and creases when the mouth is open.

Method: Lie on the back or sit upright. Use the middle finger to press and knead the Xiaguan point of the affected side for two minutes with moderate force until some tingling and distension are felt, ideally radiating all over the face.

Effect: Treat toothache, trifacial neuralgia, difficulty in opening the mouth, deviated mouth and eyes (facial paralysis), and hyposiagonarthritis.

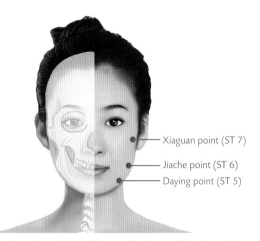

Location of the Xiaguan, Jiache and Daying points.

3. Pressing and Kneading the Jiache Point

Location: In a cavity about one cun in the upper part of the lower jaw corner, i.e. the highest point of the zygomaxillary muscle when one chews.

Method: Use the pad of the middle finger to press and knead the Jiache point of the affected side for about two minutes. Use moderate force until some tingling and distension are felt along with slight warmth and numbness as the best effect.

Effect: Treat toothache, trifacial neuralgia, problems with the masseter, difficulty in opening the mouth, freckles, chloasma, deviated mouth and eyes (facial paralysis), and excess salivating.

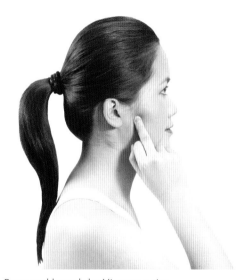

Press and knead the Xiaguan point.

4. Pressing the Daying Point

Location: In a cavity between the lip and lower jaw bone over the pulse of the facial artery.

Method: Sit upright. Use the thumb of one hand to press the Daying point from the bottom up while turning your neck to the same side.

Effect: Promote blood circulation, tighten skin, eliminate double chin and prevent facial skin from becoming loose, in addition to curing toothache and oral ulcer.

5. Pressing and Kneading the Fengchi Point

Location: In the depression on both sides of the large tendon behind the nape of the neck, next to the lower edge of the skull.

Method: Sit upright. Use the pads of the thumbs or middle fingers to press the Fengchi point on both sides, proceeding from light to heavy force. Then knead gently until some tingling and distension are felt as the best effect. In the process of massage turn the neck gently. The massage generally lasts for two minutes or so.

Effect: Cure cold, fever, neck pain, headache, dizziness, and red and swollen eyes with pain.

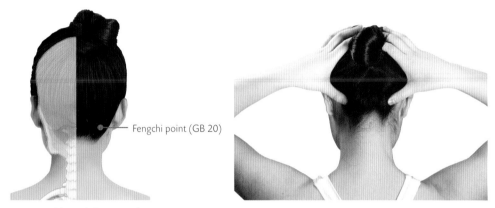

Fengchi point (GB 20)

Press and knead the Fengchi point.

6. Pressing and Kneading the Waiguan and Neiguan Points

Location: The Waiguan point is in the middle on the outside of the arm, between the ulna and radius about two cun away from the horizontal line of the wrist joint. The Neiguan point is between the two tendons about two cun above the wrist joint bend.

Method: With the front arm bent halfway, use one thumb tip to press the Waiguan point on the other arm. The index or middle finger should press the Neiguan point, pressing inward 20 to 30 times, until tingling and distension are felt.

Effect: Cure fever, cold, pneumonia, tinnitus, dumbness, stiff neck, migraine, intercostal nerve pain, upper limb joint pain, and elbow pain.

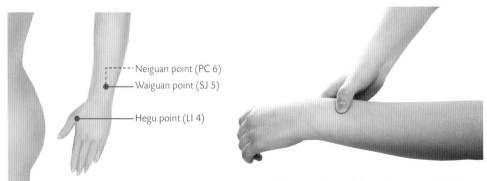

Neiguan point (PC 6)
Waiguan point (SJ 5)
Hegu point (LI 4)

Location of the Neiguan, Waiguan and Hegu points.

Press and knead the Waiguan and Neiguan points.

7. Pinching and Kneading the Hegu Point

Location: In the highest point on the back of the hand between the thumb base and the base of the index finger (in the webbing between these two fingers).

Method: Use the thumb tip of one hand to pinch the Hegu point on the other hand for about one minute, and continue pinching and kneading for about two minutes, until some tingling and distension are felt as the best effect.

Effect: Treat facioplegia, trigeminal pain, facial paralysis, deviated mouth and eyes (facial paralysis), rhinitis, headache, toothache, acne, visual fatigue, sore throat, tinnitus and hiccups.

8. Pressing and Kneading the Taixi Point

Location: In a cavity between the medial malleolus and Achilles tendon.

Method: Sit upright. Use the thumb to press and knead the Taixi point for two to three minutes until some tingling and distension are felt. This massage is prohibited during pregnancy.

Effect: Chiefly serve to cure headache, dizzy vision, stiff neck, waist tingling, tinnitus, sore throat, insomnia, frequent urination, bed-wetting, menstrual disorder, ankle swelling and pain, ankle sprain, asthma, nephritis and cystitis.

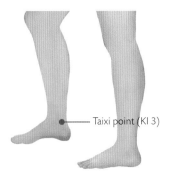
Taixi point (KI 3)

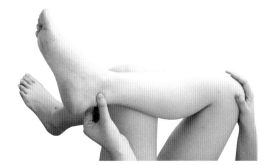

Press and knead the Taixi point.

Tips
- Pay attention to oral hygiene and form the good habit of brushing your teeth in the morning and evening. Rinse the mouth after meals.
- Timely treatment should be given to tooth decay once it is found.
- Liquor and hot food are proscribed. Avoid eating candy and cookies before going to bed.
- It is better to eat more of the foods that eliminate gastric heat and liver heat. Do not eat food that is too hard, too sour, too cold or too hot.
- Hot temper and anger can induce toothache. Therefore it is advised to be tolerant and calm.
- Keep bowels clear to prevent excrement from poisoning health.

12 | Shoulder Periarthritis

This degenerative and inflammatory disease concerns the joint capsules and soft tissues around the joints. The inflammation is not viral.

Shoulder periarthritis is often seen in people at the age of around 50. The number of female patients is slightly more than that of male patients. Most of them undertake manual labor.

If it is not treated appropriately, it may affect the functional movement of the joints and impinge on daily life. Catching a cold is often the cause of shoulder periarthritis.

Symptoms

In the early stage, there will be spasmodic pain in the shoulder joints often due to climatic changes or heavy work. Gradually it will develop into continuous pain, eventually becoming as serious as to inhibit the ability to fall asleep or to sleep on the affected side. The active and passive movements of the shoulder joints are restricted in all directions. There will be sharp pain if the shoulders are pulled. The joints may suffer from extensive pressing pain, which radiates to the neck and elbows. In addition there can be a contraction of the deltoid muscles to varying degrees.

Target Acupoints

Shoulder, back and waist: Tianzong (SI 11), Jugu (LI 6), Jianjing (GB 21).
Arms: Jianqian (SJ 14), Jianyu (LI 15), Hegu (LI 4), Jianzhen (SI 9), Quchi (LI 11), Waiguan (SJ 5).
Legs: Tiaokou (ST 38).

Recommended Massage

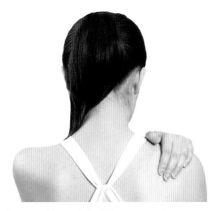
Press and knead the Tianzong point.

1. Pressing and Kneading the Tianzong Point

Location: In the depression at the center of the scapula.

Method: Sit upright and relax the neck muscles. Use the middle finger to forcefully press and knead the Tianzong point on the opposite side. Continue for two minutes until tingling and distension are felt in the shoulder and back, ideally so that weakness is felt in the arms.

Effect: Cure scapula pain, and trauma in the shoulder and back, as well as asthma.

2. Pressing and Kneading the Jugu Point

Location: In a cavity between the tip of the collarbone and the mesoscapula.

Method: Use the middle finger to press the Jugu point on the opposite side while drooping the upper arm and stretching the forearm horizontally. Press the Jugu point while extending the shoulder.

Effect: Treat shoulder periarthritis, strain of the shoulder joints and soft tissues, hematemesis, gastric bleeding, tuberculosis of neck-lymph nodes, high fever, convulsion and lower tooth pain.

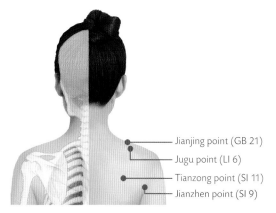

Jianjing point (GB 21)
Jugu point (LI 6)
Tianzong point (SI 11)
Jianzhen point (SI 9)

Location of the Jianjing, Jugu, Tianzong and Jianzhen points.

3. Kneading the Jianjing Point

Location: At the midpoint of the top on the shoulder.

Method: Sit upright. Use both middle fingers to press and knead the Jianjing point on both sides, with the palm heels and thenar eminences holding the upper part of the collarbone closely. The muscle in this area is lifted and pinched by the palms and fingers (with more force from the middle finger). Proceeding from light to heavy force, press, rub and knead the Jianjing point at the same time. Generally it takes

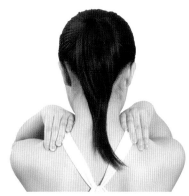

Knead the Jianjing point.

two or three minutes until you feel relaxed in the shoulders and neck. You can also do one side first and then the other side.

Effect: Treat cervical spondylosis, stiff neck, shoulder periarthritis, shoulder pain, inability to raise the arms, shoulder-back tingling and pain, sequela of apoplexy, difficult labor, fever and headache.

4. Pressing and Kneading the Jianzhen Point

Location: At the lower back of the shoulder joint.

Method: Sit upright. Use the tip of the middle finger to press and knead the Jianzhen point for two minutes with moderate force, until some tingling and distension are felt as the best effect.

Effect: Cure problems with the joints and soft tissues of the shoulder as well as upper limb paralysis and armpit sweating.

5. Pressing and Kneading the Jianqian Point

Location: At the front of the shoulder, halfway between the Jianyu point and the armpit plica.

Method: Use the pad of the thumb to press and knead the Jianqian point of the

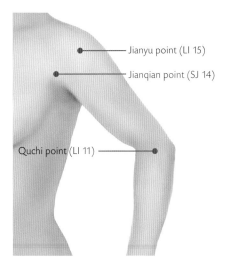

Location of the Jianyu, Jianqian and Quchi points.

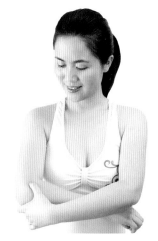

Pinch and knead the Quchi point.

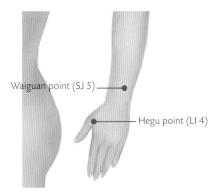

Location of the Waiguan and Hegu points.

affected side for two minutes with moderate force, until some tingling and distension are felt as the best effect.

Effect: Cure shoulder-arm pain and difficulty in raising the arm.

6. Pinching and Pressing the Jianyu Point

Location: In a cavity just before the shoulder peak when one raises the upper arm horizontally.

Method: Sit upright. Use the index finger to press the Jianyu point while using the thumb to press the Jianqian point, repeating 30 to 50 times.

Effect: Prevent and cure cervical spondylosis, shoulder periarthritis, scapula pain, arm pain, upper limb paralysis and shoulder-arm rheumatalgia.

7. Pinching and Kneading the Quchi Point

Location: With the elbow bent halfway, on the outer side of the cubital transverse crease.

Method: Sit upright with the arm bent halfway. Use the thumb of the other hand to pinch and press the Quchi point for one minute. Then press and knead for another two minutes, until some tingling and distension are felt.

Effect: Treat all kinds of symptoms of fever, headache resulting from high blood pressure, red face and eyes, sore throat, toothache, acne, hives, erysipelas and arm pain.

8. Pinching and Kneading the Hegu Point

Location: In the highest point on the back of the hand between the thumb base and the base of the index finger (in the webbing between these two fingers).

Method: Use the thumb tip of one hand to pinch the Hegu point on the other hand for about one minute, and continue pinching and kneading for about two minutes, until some tingling and distension are felt as the best effect.

Effect: Treat facioplegia, trigeminal pain, facial paralysis, deviated mouth and eyes (facial paralysis), rhinitis, headache, toothache, acne, visual fatigue, sore throat, tinnitus and hiccups.

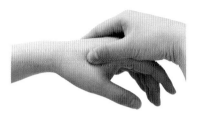

Pinch and knead the Hegu point.

9. Pressing and Kneading the Waiguan Point

Location: In the middle on the outside of the arm, between the ulna and radius about two cun away from the horizontal line of the wrist joint.

Method: With the forearm bent halfway, use the pad of the thumb on the healthy side of the body to forcefully press the Waiguan point of the affected side. Move for two minutes, until some tingling and distension are felt, ideally radiating numbness to the palm and fingers.

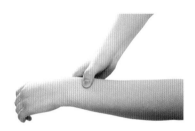

Press and knead the Waiguan point.

Effect: Cure fever, cold, pneumonia, tinnitus, dumbness, stiff neck, migraine, intercostal nerve pain, upper limb joint pain, and elbow pain.

10. Pressing and Kneading the Tiaokou Point

Location: At the posterior shank, two centimeters outside the tibial crest, on the midpoint of the line connecting the small bone protruding under the knee and the outer ankle.

Method: Sit upright. Use the middle or index finger to press and knead the Tiaokou point 20 to 40 times, proceeding from light to heavy force, until some tingling and distension are felt.

Effect: Cure shoulder periarthritis, shoulder pain, cold feeling, pain and swelling of the shanks.

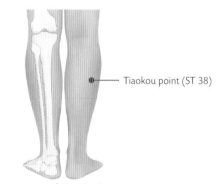

Tiaokou point (ST 38)

Location of the Tiaokou point.

Tips
- Pay attention to nutrition, making sure you get appropriate vitamins and minerals.
- Be sure to keep warm to protect the shoulders from chill.
- If you already are affected, undergo timely treatment.
- Keep exercising the shoulder muscles to prevent and delay the occurrence and development of shoulder periarthritis. Research has shown that among people with strong shoulder muscles, the incidence of shoulder periarthritis decreases by 80 percent.

13 | Shoulder-Neck Fasciitis

Also called muscular rheumatism, it generally refers to non-viral inflammation in such soft tissues as the fascia, muscles, tendons and ligaments leading to symptoms including shoulder-back pain, stiffness, restricted movement and weakness.

Symptoms

Extensive tingling and pain in the neck, shoulders and back accompanied by a sense of heaviness, numbness, stiffness and restriction of movement. Such tingling and pain can radiate to the rear of the head and upper arms.

The pain attacks continuously and may become worse due to infection, fatigue, cold and dampness.

Physical examination can reveal the strain in the neck muscles, and the pressure pain point is often felt in the spinous process (the bony projection on the back of the vertebrae) as well as the trapezius and rhomboideus. The pressure pain is limited to the pain point instead of radiating along the direction of the nerves.

Fasciitis of the neck and shoulder muscles attacks slowly over a long time. Examination by X-ray mostly results in negative findings.

Target Acupoints

Shoulder, back and waist: Jianjing (GB 21), Fengmen (BL 12), Tianzong (SI 11), Bingfeng (SI 12), Quyuan (SI 13), Jianwaishu (SI 14), Dazhui (DU 14).

Recommended Massage

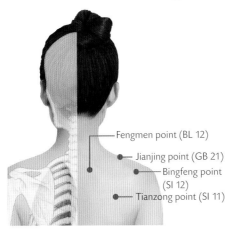

Location of the Jianjing, Fengmen, Bingfeng and Tianzong points.

— Fengmen point (BL 12)
— Jianjing point (GB 21)
— Bingfeng point (SI 12)
— Tianzong point (SI 11)

1. Kneading the Jianjing Point
Location: At the midpoint of the top on the shoulder.

Method: Sit upright. Use both middle fingers to press and knead the Jianjing point on both sides, with the palm heels and thenar eminences holding the upper part of the collarbone closely. The muscle in this area is lifted and pinched by the palms and fingers (with more force from the middle finger). Proceeding from light to heavy force, press, rub and knead the Jianjing point at the same time. Generally it takes two or three minutes until you feel relaxed in the shoulders and neck. You can also do one side first and then the other side.

Effect: Treat cervical spondylosis, stiff neck, shoulder periarthritis, shoulder pain, inability to raise the arms, shoulder-back tingling and pain, sequela of apoplexy, difficult labor, fever and headache.

2. Pressing and Kneading the Fengmen Point
Location: 1.5 cun below the spinous process of the second thoracic vertebra.

Method: Sit upright. Use the tip of the middle finger of the left hand to press and knead the Fengmen point of the right side. At the same time use the tip of the right middle finger to press and knead the Fengmen point on the left. Continue for two minutes until some tingling and distension are obvious.

Effect: Chiefly serve to cure severe neck-back pain, cold and diseases of the respiratory system.

3. Pressing and Kneading the Tianzong Point
Location: In the depression at the center of the scapula.

Method: Sit upright. Relax the neck muscles and then use the middle finger to press, rub and knead the Tianzong point forcefully until you feel tingling and distension in the shoulder, and back and weakness in the arms.

Effect: Cure scapula pain, and trauma in the shoulder and back, as well as asthma.

4. Pressing and Kneading the Bingfeng Point
Location: In a cavity that appears when the arm is raised, right above the Tianzong point in the middle of the supraspinal fossa of the scapula.

Method: Sit upright. Use the index, middle and ring finger to press and knead the Bingfeng point of the affected side. Continue for two minutes, until tingling and distension are felt in the shoulder and back; ideally weakness should be felt in the upper limbs.

Effect: Chiefly serve to cure scapula pain, tingling and numbness of the upper limbs, and ailments of the scapula and upper limbs.

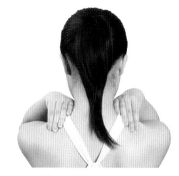
Press and knead the Jianjing point.

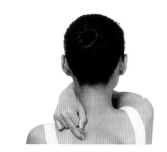
Press and knead the Fengmen point.

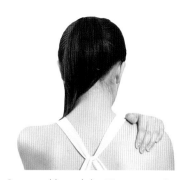
Press and knead the Tianzong point.

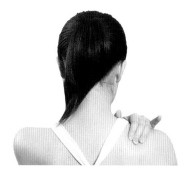
Press and knead the Bingfeng point.

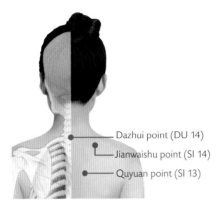

Location of the Dazhui, Jianwaishu and Quyuan points.

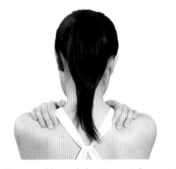

Press and knead the Jianwaishu point.

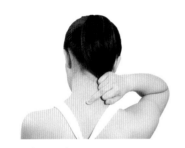

Press the Dazhui point.

5. Pressing the Quyuan Point

Location: By the top inner corner of the scapula, in a cavity.

Method: Use the index or middle finger to press the Quyuan point. Repeat 30 to 40 times, enabling the body to feel a relaxed and stabilizing mood.

Effect: Chiefly serve to cure scapula pain.

6. Pressing and Kneading the Jianwaishu Point

Location: Three cun beside the spinous process of the first thoracic vertebra.

Method. Use the tips of the middle fingers to press and knead the Jianwaishu point of both sides for two minutes. The left hand will work on the right Jianwaishu point and vice versa. Use slightly heavy force until tingling and distension are obvious. The back should feel relaxed after massage.

Effect: Chiefly serve to cure shoulder-back pain, severe neck pain and other kinds of shoulder, back and neck pain.

7. Pressing the Dazhui Point

Location: Under the spinous process of the seventh cervical vertebrae.

Method: Sit on a chair. Use the middle finger to press the Dazhui point while extending the elbow and leaning backward.

Effect: Reduce inner heat, relieve exterior syndrome, help to prevent malaria and dysentery, and treat cold, fever, chill, nasal congestion, cough, neck pain and acne.

Tips

- Do not lower the head for a long time while working.
- If it is unavoidable, one must move around after working in such a posture for 20 or 30 minutes, for instance, stretching the arms, rotating the head, or supporting the waist with the hands and bending the neck to look upward. Exercise for no less than three minutes each time.

14 | Waist-Back Pain

Quite common among people these days, this is chronic or acute inflammation of the muscles or fascia due to staying in one position for a long time or trauma in the waist.

In addition infiltration of cold wind into the waist and back is also apt to cause such pain. Psoatic strain, lumbar disc herniation, waist-back fasciitis and waist sprain may be connected with either waist or back pain.

Waist-back pain can be eased through rest. It attacks more sharply after work, and sitting or standing for a long time can also make it worse. Some patients cannot even bend down to pick up things and their breathing may be impinged.

Symptoms

According to the symptoms, it can be divided into two types: 1) waist-back pain with lower limb pain or numbness and 2) simple waist-back pain.

The first type is mostly caused by the fact that the spinal cords along the chest and waist, or cauda equine nerve or nerve roots and trunks, are pressed and irritated.

Simple waist-back pain refers to a condition free from lower limb pain or numbness, with several cases as follows:

• Tingling and pain on both sides of the spine in the waist and back: Bending down or sitting for a long time will make it worse, but it will ease after lying down or moving around a little.

• Pain at the center of the waist and back: Patients will feel less pain, or none, when standing straight, but feel more pain and weakness in the waist when bending forward. If such pain attacks the chest and waist, it is mostly supraspinal desmitis. If the pain attacks the waist only, it is mostly interspinous desmitis.

• Sudden pain when moving upright after bending down: If the case quickly becomes more serious, leading to stiff waist, it is mostly due to the synovium being inserted into the joint.

Target Acupoints

Shoulder, back, waist and buttocks: Xinshu (BL 15), Zhiyang (DU 9), Ganshu (BL 18), Weishu (BL 21), Geshu (BL 17), Baliao (BL 31–34), Shenshu (BL 23), Zhibian (BL 54), Zhishi (BL 52), Dachangshu (BL 25), Yaoyan (EX-B 7), Huantiao (GB 30).
Chest and abdomen: Danzhong (RN 17), Tianshu (ST 25).
Legs: Weizhong (BL 40), Chengshan (BL 57), Chengfu (BL 36), Chengjin (BL 56).

Recommended Massage

1. Pressing the Xinshu Point
Location: Under the fifth thoracic vertebra on the inner side of the scapula, 1.5 cun horizontally away.

Method: Sit on a chair. Use the middle finger to press and knead the Xinshu point for about two minutes, until tingling and distension are felt.

Effect: Treat agitation, palpitation, difficulty breathing, heart pain, cough, hematemesis, chest-back pain, insomnia, forgetfulness, night sweating, wet dream and epilepsy.

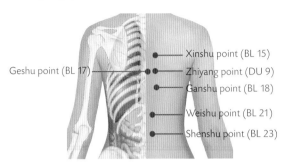

Geshu point (BL 17)
Xinshu point (BL 15)
Zhiyang point (DU 9)
Ganshu point (BL 18)
Weishu point (BL 21)
Shenshu point (BL 23)

Location of the Xinshu, Zhiyang, Geshu, Ganshu, Weishu and Shenshu points.

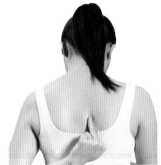

Press the Xinshu point.

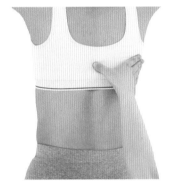

Press the Zhiyang point.

2. Pressing the Zhiyang Point

Location: In a cavity below the spinous process of the seventh thoracic vertebra on the midline of the back.

Method: Lie down. Use the thumb to press the Zhiyang point for about two minutes.

Effect: Treat chest pain, waist-back pain, jaundice, cholecystitis (inflammation of gallbladder), ascariasis (parasitic infection) of the biliary tract, gastroenteritis and intercostal nerve pain.

3. Pressing and Kneading the Ganshu Point

Location: 1.5 cun away from the ninth thoracic spinal process on the inner side of the scapula.

Method: Sit upright. Use the four knuckles to press and knead the Ganshu point while moving down forcefully for about two minutes, until some tingling and distension are felt as the best effect.

Effect: Treat distension and pain of both sides of the chest, breast pain with swelling, waist-back pain, agitation, irritability, indigestion and aversion to food, neurasthenia, hepatitis, jaundice (icterus), nausea, vomiting, lack of appetite and dizziness.

4. Pressing and Kneading the Weishu Point

Location: About 1.5 cun below the spinous process of the twelfth thoracic vertebra.

Method: Sit or stand. Use the middle fingers to press and knead the Weishu point of both sides (with the thumb against the ribs) forcefully for two minutes.

Alternately make a fist and use the protruding index knuckle to press and knead it for two minutes. Or with a loose fist, press and rub the point for two minutes. In all cases some tingling and distension are felt as the best effect.

Effect: Treat all kinds of diseases and symptoms of the digestive system, such as acute gastritis, chronic gastritis, gastroptosis, stomach atony, abdominal distension, abdominal pain, lack of appetite, nausea and vomiting.

5. Pressing the Geshu Point

Location: At the point 1.5 cun away from the spinous process of the seventh thoracic vertebra.

Method: Sit upright. Use the middle fingers to press forcefully for about two minutes.

Effect: Serve to clear the lungs, stop vomiting, promote the circulation of blood and vital energy, and to treat back pain due to blood congestion, sprain of the back muscle, chronic bleeding diseases, prolonged lochiorrhea after giving birth, dizziness resulting from low blood pressure, anemia, hiccups, nervous vomiting, hives and skin diseases.

6. Pressing and Kneading the Shenshu Point

Location: 1.5 cun horizontally from the second lumbar spinal process.

Method: Lie on the back or sit upright. Use the two middle fingers to forcefully press and knead the Shenshu point of both sides 30 to 50 times, keeping the thumbs by the ribs. Or, with a clenched fist, use the knuckle of the index finger to press and knead the Shenshu point 30 to 50 times. You might also try using a loose fist to knead and rub 30 to 50 times, until some warmth is felt as the best effect.

Effect: Treat waist tingling and leg pain, lumbar muscle strain, lumbar disc herniation, leg swelling, fatigue all over the body, impotence, nocturnal emission, premature ejaculation and menstrual disorder.

7. Kneading and Rubbing the Baliao Points

Location: There are eight Baliao points in total, four on each side of the sacral spine. These are the upper, secondary, middle and lower Baliao points. They are located respectively in the first, second, third and fourth posterior sacral foramina (opening between vertebrae).

Method: Sit upright. Use the palm to knead, or rub up and down, along the sacral vertebrae for about two minutes, until some tingling and distension are felt as the best effect.

Effect: Cure pain in the lumbosacral spine, constipation, distension and pain in the lower abdomen, pelvic inflammation, difficult urination, menstrual disorder and hemorrhoids.

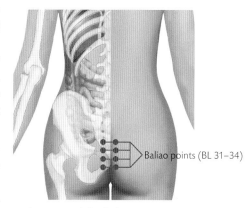

Baliao points (BL 31–34)

Location of the Baliao points.

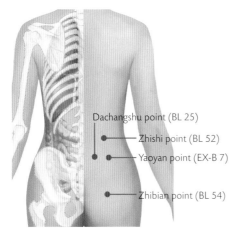

Location of the Zhishi, Dachangshu, Yaoyan and Zhibian points.

Dachangshu point (BL 25)
Zhishi point (BL 52)
Yaoyan point (EX-B 7)
Zhibian point (BL 54)

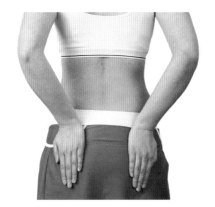

Press and knead the Zhibian point.

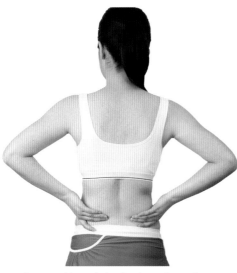

Press and knead the Dachangshu point.

8. Pressing and Kneading the Zhibian Point

Location: Three cun away from the median sacral crest.

Method: In a standing position, use both palm heels to press and knead the Zhibian point outward for two to three minutes, until some tingling and distension are felt as the best effect.

Effect: Cure waist-back pain, leg pain, constipation, hemorrhoids, difficult urination and vaginal pain.

9. Pressing the Zhishi Point

Location: Three cun away from the spinous process of the second lumbar vertebra.

Method: Kneel and use the thumb to press the Zhishi point on the same side, while leaning to the same side as the point being pressed.

Effect: Treat nocturnal emission, impotence, difficult urination, edema, waist-back tingling and pain, lumbar muscle strain, sciatica, testicular swelling, pain, vaginal pain, indigestion, nausea and vomiting.

10. Pressing and Kneading the Dachangshu Point

Location: About 1.5 cun away from the fourth lumbar vertebra on two sides.

Method: Sit or stand with hands akimbo. Use the pad of the middle finger to forcefully press and knead the Dachangshu point on both sides for about two minutes. Alternatively you can make a fist and use the knuckle of the index finger to press for one minute, until some warmth or tingling and distension are felt as the best effect.

Effect: Treat constipation, abdominal pain, abdominal distension, diarrhea, borborygmus, waist-back pain and premature ejaculation.

11. Pressing and Kneading the Yaoyan Point

Location: At the point 3.5 cun away from the spinous process of the fourth lumbar vertebra.

Method: Sit or stand. Make a fist and use the knuckle of the middle finger to press and knead the point with moderate force until warmth, tingling and distension are felt as the best effect.

Effect: Chiefly serve to cure sprain of soft tissues of the waist, lumbar bone hyperplasia, lumbar disc herniation, urinary incontinence, urinary retention, nephroptosis, menstrual disorder and leukorrhagia.

12. Pressing and Kneading the Huantiao Point

Location: In the depression on the outer side of the gluteus maximus, on both sides when standing.

Method: Lie on your side (with the lower leg stretched and upper leg bent) or on the back. Use the thumb or middle finger to press and knead the point forcefully, 20 to 30 times, until some tingling and distension are felt or a feeling of electric shock is radiated to the lower limbs.

Effect: Cure and prevent sciatica, paralysis of the lower limbs, inflammation of the hip, and sprain of surrounding soft tissues.

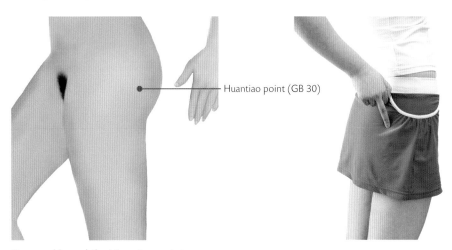

Huantiao point (GB 30)

Press and knead the Huantiao point.

13. Pressing the Danzhong Point

Location: Directly in the middle of the chest between the nipples.

Method: Sit upright. Use the thenar eminence to press the point for about three minutes while leaning backward.

Effect: Cure difficulty in breathing, cough, chest pain, hyperplasia of the mammary glands, breast pain, agalactia (lactation difficulty), palpitation and obesity.

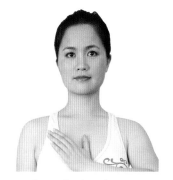

Press the Danzhong point.

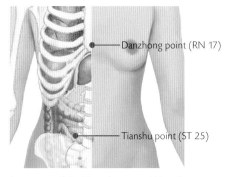

Location of the Danzhong and Tianshu points.

14. Pressing and Kneading the Tianshu Point

Location: About two cun horizontally away from the navel.

Method: Lie on the back. Use the index fingers to press and knead the point for about three minutes, making small circles.

Effect: Channel the circulation of blood and vital energy, as well as adjust menstruation and stop pain. It has a good effect on curing gastric and intestinal diseases and diseases of the liver, gallbladder and spleen, particularly chronic gastritis coupled with nausea and vomiting as well as chronic diarrhea. It is also beneficial in cases of diseases concerned with the uterus, ovary and fallopian tube.

15. Plucking the Chengfu Point

Location: At the center of the gluteal fold, where the buttock meets the upper leg.

Method: While standing, use the index, middle and ring finger to press the Chengfu point, plucking it from inward to outward for two minutes, until tingling and distension are felt as the best effect.

Effect: Cure waist and buttock pain, sciatica, drooping buttocks, underdeveloped muscle of the buttocks and hemorrhoids.

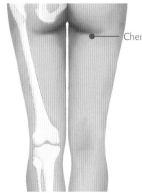

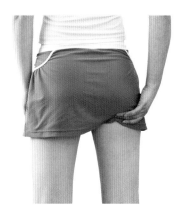

Pluck the Chengfu point.

16. Pressing and Kneading the Weizhong Point

Location: Right in the middle of popliteal crease (at the back of the knee).

Method: Sit upright. Use the middle or index finger to press the Weizhong point of the affected side, keeping the thumb pressing just outside the patella. Proceed from light to heavy force, repeating 20 to 40 times.

Effect: Cure all kinds of waist-back pain, tingling in the waist, pain and swelling in the legs, pain around the knee joints, and paralysis of the lower limbs. It also eases fatigue all over the body.

17. Pressing the Chengshan Point

Location: In a cavity in the middle of the rear of the lower leg, at the top of the depression between the two muscles of the calf.

Method: Sit upright. Use the thumb to press the Chengshan point for one minute, until some tingling and distension are felt as the best effect.

Effect: Treat waist-back pain, sciatica, spasm of the gastrocnemius muscle in the calf, leg paralysis, thickening in the lower leg, and constipation.

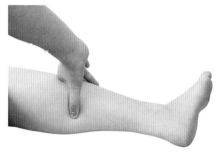

Press the Chengshan point.

18. Pressing and Kneading the Chengjin Point

Location: In the middle of the gastrocnemius muscle; or on the highest prominence of the calf muscle if lying down or sitting upright with the foot slack.

Method: Sitting cross-legged, hold up one knee, fixed by one hand, while using the full surface of the thumb of the other hand to press and knead the Chengjin point in a circular manner. You can also use the thumb to press and knead the Chengjin point of the affected side clockwise for two minutes, proceeding from light to heavy force, until tingling and distension are felt as the best effect.

Effect: Chiefly serves to cure waist and leg spasm, pain and hemorrhoids.

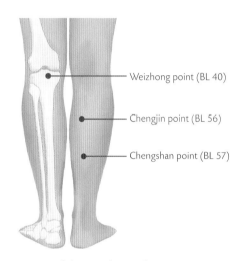

Weizhong point (BL 40)

Chengjin point (BL 56)

Chengshan point (BL 57)

Location of the Weizhong, Chengjin and Chengshan points.

Tips

Do not neglect the possibility of the waist-back pain being ankylosing spondylitis (spinal arthritis). It is mostly seen in males from 15 to 40, with the age of 20 being the peak period.

Its early-stage symptom is not typical. There will be waist-back pain at the beginning, which will quickly improve after the patient moves around a bit. This means it is often overlooked.

In addition the patient will suffer from stiffness in the morning, sometimes lasting for several hours. Such stiffness is more obvious for those who seldom exercise, and they may have to roll down from bed to get up.

If young and middle-aged patients suffer from waist-back pain for three consecutive months, as well as blunt pain in the morning or after sitting for a long time, they should see a doctor, preferably in the analgesic department or specializing in rheumatism and immunity, for timely examination.

15 | Acute Lumbar Sprain

This is acute wrenching or tearing caused by sudden and excessive pull of outer force in such soft tissues as the lumbar muscles, fascia and ligaments. It often takes place when people lift heavy things as their lumbar muscles contract forcefully at the same time, leading to forced strain in the point of attachment of the soft tissues.

Symptoms

It is chiefly marked by pain at waist level and restriction over body movement. Chinese medicine calls it "sudden waist sprain" or "qi disorder." The patients might even have heard a clear breaking sound at the time of injury. Those who suffer sharp lumbar pain cannot move around at all. Those with less serious cases can still work, but may suffer greater pain after a period of rest, even to the extent of failing to get up from bed the following day.

The midsection of the patient will be stiff in examination along with the disappearance of the lumbar convex, the natural lateral curvature of the spinal column, as well as possible spasm of the sacral spinal muscle. Obvious pressure pain points can be found at the area of trauma.

Target Acupoints

Head and neck: Renzhong (DU 26).
Shoulder, back, waist and buttocks: Pain point, Huantiao (GB 30), Yaoyan (EX-B 7), Baliao(BL 31–34).
Arms: Lumbar pain point.
Chest and abdomen: Daju (ST 27).
Legs: Weizhong (BL 40), Kunlun (BL 60).

Recommended Massage

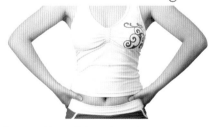
Press and knead the pain point.

1. Pressing and Kneading the Pain Point
Location: Pain point of the sprain.

Method: Choose the most comfortable posture. Use the four fingers to press and knead the point for three to five minutes, proceeding from light to heavy force.

Effect: Ease pain.

2. Pressing and Kneading the Huantiao Point
Location: In the depression on the outer side of the gluteus maximus, on both sides when standing.

Method: Lie on your side (with the lower leg stretched and upper leg bent) or on the back. Use the thumb or middle finger to press and knead the point forcefully, 20 to 30 times, until some tingling and distension are felt or a feeling of electric shock is radiated to the lower limbs.

Effect: Cure and prevent sciatica, paralysis of the lower limbs, inflammation of the hip, and sprain of surrounding soft tissues.

3. Pressing and Kneading the Yaoyan Point

Location: At the point 3.5 cun away from the spinous process of the fourth lumbar vertebra.

Method: Sit or stand. Make a fist and use the knuckle of the middle finger to press and knead the point with moderate force until warmth, tingling and distension are felt as the best effect.

Effect: Chiefly serve to cure sprain of soft tissues of the waist, lumbar bone hyperplasia, lumbar disc herniation, urinary incontinence, urinary retention, nephroptosis, menstrual disorder and leukorrhagia.

4. Kneading and Rubbing the Baliao Points

Location: There are eight Baliao points in total, four on each side of the sacral spine. These are the upper, secondary, middle and lower Baliao points. They are located respectively in the first, second, third and fourth posterior sacral foramina (opening between vertebrae).

Method: Sit upright. Use the palm to knead, or rub up and down, along the sacral vertebrae for about two minutes, until some tingling and distension are felt as the best effect.

Effect: Cure pain in the lumbosacral spine, constipation, distension and pain in the lower abdomen, pelvic inflammation, difficult urination, menstrual disorder and hemorrhoids.

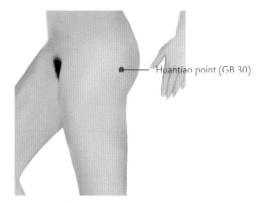

Location of the Huantiao point.

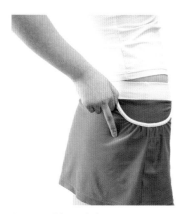

Press and knead the Yaoyan point.

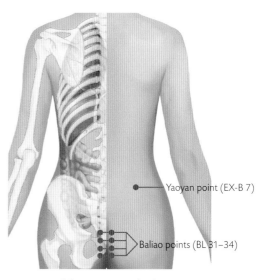

Location of the Yaoyan and Baliao points.

5. Pressing and Pinching the Renzhong Point

Location: In the middle of the groove below the nose, between the lip and the nose.

   Method: Lie on the back. Use the thumb tip to press and pinch the Renzhong point for one minute with somewhat heavy force, until tingling and distension are felt as the best effect.

   Effect: Raise blood pressure, influence breathing and benefit rhythmic respiration, as well as treat unconsciousness, angina, severe waist-back pain and difficulty in breathing.

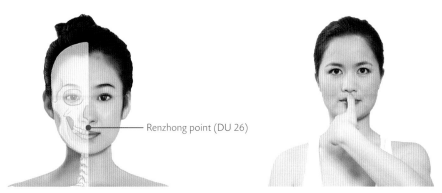

Renzhong point (DU 26)

Press and pinch the Renzhong point.

6. Pressing the Lumbar Pain Point

Location: Two spots on the back of each hand, one is between the second and third metacarpal bone, while the other is between the fourth and fifth metacarpal bone (totaling four in the body).

   Method: While standing use the thumb tip to press the pain point for two to three minutes, until tingling and distension are felt, alternating between two hands. In the course of massage move the waist around.

   Effect: Treat acute lumbar sprain.

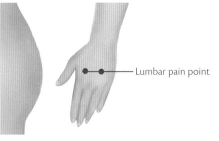

Lumbar pain point

Location of the lumber pain point.

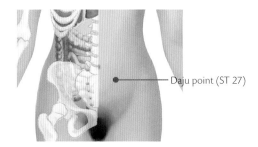

Daju point (ST 27)

Location of the Daju point.

7. Pressing and Kneading the Daju Point

Location: Two cun below the navel, two cun away from the median line.

   Method: Lie on the back with knees bent. Using the four fingers of both hands, press and knead it respectively.

   Effect: Chiefly serve to cure distension of the lower abdomen, difficult urination, hernia, nocturnal emission, premature ejaculation, convulsion of the rectus abdominis, intestinal obstruction, cystitis and urinary retention.

8. Pressing and Kneading the Weizhong Point

Location: Right in the middle of popliteal crease (at the back of the knee).

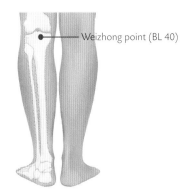
Weizhong point (BL 40)

Method: Sit upright. Use the middle or index finger to press the Weizhong point of the affected side, keeping the thumb pressing just outside the patella. Proceed from light to heavy force, repeating 20 to 40 times.

Effect: Cure all kinds of waist-back pain, tingling in the waist, pain and swelling in the legs, pain around the knee joints, and paralysis of the lower limbs.

Location of the Weizhong point.

9. Pressing the Kunlun Point

Location: In a cavity directly in the rear of the lateral malleolus.

Method: Kneel on one knee only. Use the thumb to press the Kunlun point of the same side for about three minutes.

Effect: Cure ankle sprain, pain with swelling, high blood pressure, insomnia, forgetfulness, menstrual disorder, nocturnal emission, impotence, pain during sexual intercourse, and frequent urination.

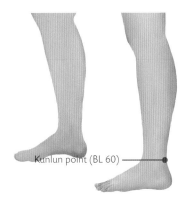
Kunlun point (BL 60)

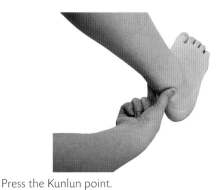
Press the Kunlun point.

Tips

If you experience "sudden waist sprain," see a doctor as soon as possible for timely and proper treatment. Patients should be sure to rest; it is preferable to sleep with a wood platform under the mattress. A box spring is too soft, which will result in the lateral curvature of the spinal column, worsening the lumbar illness.

16 Lumbar Muscle Strain

This is due to ineffective treatment of acute lumbar sprain, incomplete recovery from lumbar injury or repeated minor injuries. It mostly occurs among adults. The condition can be associated with remaining in a fixed position for a long time or having undesirable posture, which can lead to repeated attacks.

Symptoms

There is pain in a large area of one side or both sides of the waist, chiefly marked by tingling and pain. With a pressure pain point in the waist, there are no unusual phenomena in the outer waist or obvious lumbar muscle spasm. Lumbar activities are unrestricted except in a few cases where there is slight restriction.

The strain becomes more severe when one feels tired at work, and it diminishes when one rests. Although pain is absent or tolerable when one gets up in the morning, it becomes painful at night. Moving around adequately or often changing body position reduces the pain, but excessive activities make it severe. The patient cannot bend to work, but adjusting the body position and straightening up while supporting the hips with the hands can ease the pain.

Target Acupoints

Shoulder, back, waist and buttocks: Shenshu (BL 23), Yaoyan (EX-B 7), third transverse process of the waist, Baliao (BL 31–34), Zhibian (BL 54), Huantiao (GB 30), Juliao (GB 29).
Legs: Weizhong (BL 40).

Recommended Massage

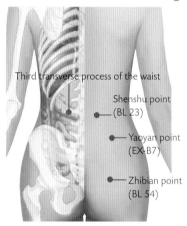

Location of the third transverse process point and the Shenshu, Yaoyan and Zhibian points.

Third transverse process of the waist

Shenshu point (BL 23)

Yaoyan point (EX-B7)

Zhibian point (BL 54)

1. Pressing and Kneading the Shenshu Point
Location: 1.5 cun horizontally from the second lumbar spinal process.

Method: Lie on the back or sit upright. Use the two middle fingers to forcefully press and knead the Shenshu point of both sides 30 to 50 times, keeping the thumbs by the ribs. Or, with a clenched fist, use the knuckle of the index finger to press and knead the Shenshu point 30 to 50 times. You might also try using a loose fist to knead and rub 30 to 50 times, until some warmth is felt as the best effect.

Effect: Treat waist tingling and leg pain, lumbar muscle strain, lumbar disc herniation, leg swelling, fatigue all over the body, impotence, nocturnal emission, premature ejaculation and menstrual disorder.

2. Pressing and Kneading the Yaoyan Point

Location: At the point 3.5 cun away from the spinous process of the fourth lumbar vertebra.

Method: Sit or stand. Make a fist and use the knuckle of the middle finger to press and knead the point with moderate force until warmth, tingling and distension are felt as the best effect.

Effect: Chiefly serve to cure sprain of soft tissues of the waist, lumbar bone hyperplasia, lumbar disc herniation, urinary incontinence, urinary retention, nephroptosis, menstrual disorder and leukorrhagia.

3. Kneading the Third Transverse Process

Location: At the transverse process (small bony projection off the sides) of the third lumbar vertebra.

Method: Sit upright. Use a clenched fist to knead it for three minutes, until tingling and distension are obviously felt with slight warmth as the best effect.

Effect: Ease pain and relax adhesion.

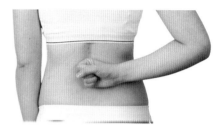

Knead the third transverse process.

4. Pressing and Kneading the Zhibian Point

Location: Three cun away from the median sacral crest.

Method: In a standing position, use both palm heels to press and knead the Zhibian point outward for two to three minutes, until some tingling and distension are felt as the best effect.

Effect: Cure waist-back pain, leg pain, constipation, hemorrhoids, difficult urination and vaginal pain.

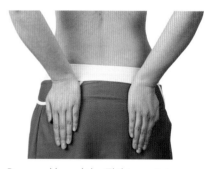

Press and knead the Zhibian point.

5. Kneading and Rubbing the Baliao Points

Location: There are eight Baliao points in total, four on each side of the sacral spine. These are the upper, secondary, middle and lower Baliao points. They are located respectively in the first, second, third and fourth posterior sacral foramina (opening between vertebrae).

Method: Sit upright. Use the palm to knead, or rub up and down, along the sacral vertebrae for about two minutes, until some tingling and distension are felt as the best effect.

Effect: Cure pain in the lumbosacral spine, constipation, distension and pain in the lower abdomen, pelvic inflammation, difficult urination, menstrual disorder and hemorrhoids.

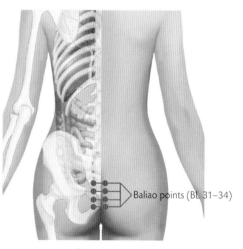

Baliao points (BL 31–34)

Location of the Baliao points.

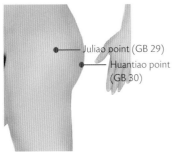

Location of the Juliao and Huantiao points.

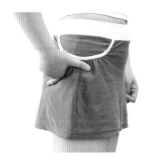

Push and press the Juliao point.

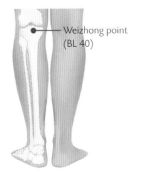

Location of the Weizhong point.

6. Pressing and Kneading the Huantiao Point

Location: In the depression on the outer side of the gluteus maximus, on both sides when standing.

Method: Lie on your side (with the lower leg stretched and upper leg bent) or on the back. Use the thumb or middle finger to press and knead the point forcefully, 20 to 30 times, until some tingling and distension are felt or a feeling of electric shock is radiated to the lower limbs.

Effect: Cure and prevent sciatica, paralysis of the lower limbs, inflammation of the hip, and sprain of surrounding soft tissues.

7. Pushing and Pressing the Juliao Point

Location: In the middle between the anterior superior iliac vertebra and the most protruding point of the greater trochanter of the femur.

Method: While standing, use the thumb tip to forcefully push the Juliao point, proceeding from light to heavy force for two to three minutes continuously.

Effect: Cure waist-leg pain, paralysis, flaccid leg muscles and hernia.

8. Pressing and Kneading the Weizhong Point

Location: Right in the middle of popliteal crease (at the back of the knee).

Method: Sit upright. Use the middle or index finger to press the Weizhong point of the affected side, keeping the thumb pressing just outside the patella. Proceed from light to heavy force, repeating 20 to 40 times.

Effect: Cure all kinds of waist-back pain, tingling in the waist, pain and swelling in the legs, pain around the knee joints, and paralysis of the lower limbs. It also eases fatigue all over the body.

Tips

- Avoid environments that are cold and damp or damp and hot.
- Do not sit or lie on the damp ground. Do not walk in rain or wade across the water. Dry the body and change clothes in a timely manner after sweating.
- Avoiding working in an undesirable posture for a long duration. Those who must maintain a set posture during working should persist in physical exercise.
- Recommended exercise: With arms akimbo, stand with legs shoulder-width apart and relax at the waist. Breathe evenly and rotate at the waist. Proceed gradually from a small to a large circle, revolving 80 to 100 times generally.

17 | Sciatica

It is caused by pathological changes in the sciatic nerve that controls the legs. The pain syndrome extends along the sciatic nerve (the waist, buttocks, rear of thighs, rear outer side of lower legs, and outer side of feet).

It is mostly seen in one side among young and middle-aged males. The intensity and duration of the pain are associated with its cause and degree of urgency.

Symptoms

There are two kinds of sciatica with different symptoms:

Nerve root sciatica: The pain often radiates from the waist to one side of the buttocks, the rear of the thigh, and the outer side of the lower leg and foot, with a feeling of burning or knife-like pain. Such pain becomes severe when one coughs or exerts force, and is even more severe at night. There is numbness and loss of feeling in the outer calf or foot dorsum. There are various causes of nerve root sciatica. The most common is lumbar disc herniation. Often exerting force, bending down or doing strenuous exercises can also lead to sciatica.

Nerve trunk sciatica: The pain often radiates from the buttocks to the rear of the buttocks, the rear outer side of the lower legs and outside of the feet. The pain will be more severe when one walks, moves around and exerts the sciatic nerve. In addition the spine may bend toward the affected side to reduce the pull on the sciatic nerve trunks.

Target Acupoints

Shoulder, back, waist and buttocks: Zhibian (BL 54), Dachangshu (BL 25), Huantiao (GB 30), Juliao (GB 29).
Legs: Chengfu (BL 36), Yanglingquan (GB 34), Weizhong (BL 40), Chengshan (BL 57), Kunlun (BL 60), Weiyang (BL 39), Yinmen (BL 37).

Recommended Massage

1. Pressing and Kneading the Zhibian Point
Location: Three cun away from the median sacral crest.

Method: In a standing position, use both palm heels to press and knead the Zhibian point outward for two to three minutes, until some tingling and distension are felt as the best effect.

Effect: Cure waist-back pain, leg pain, constipation, hemorrhoids, difficult urination and vaginal pain.

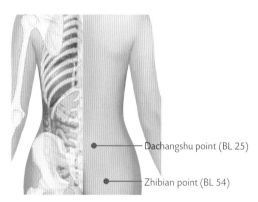

Dachangshu point (BL 25)

Zhibian point (BL 54)

Location of the Dachangshu and Zhibian points.

2. Pressing the Dachangshu Point

Location: About 1.5 cun away from the fourth lumbar vertebra on two sides.

Method: Lie on the back with knees bent. Use the protruding part of clenched fists to forcefully press Dachangshu point, taking advantage of the weight. You can also sit or stand with arms akimbo. Use the pad of the middle finger to forcefully press and knead the Dachangshu point on both sides for about two minutes. Or make a fist and use the knuckle of the index finger, pressing it for one minute, until some tingling and distension are felt as the best effect.

Effect: Cure constipation, abdominal pain and distension, diarrhea, borborygmus, waist-back pain and premature ejaculation.

3. Pushing and Pressing the Juliao Point

Location: In the middle between the anterior superior iliac vertebra and the most protruding point of the greater trochanter of the femur.

Method: Sit upright. Use the thumb tip to forcefully push the Juliao point, proceeding from light to heavy force for two to three minutes continuously.

Effect: Cure waist-leg pain, paralysis, flaccid leg muscles and hernia.

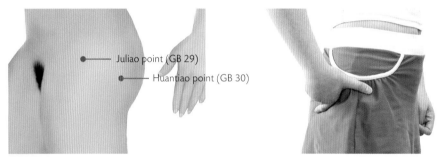

Location of the Juliao and Huantiao points.   Push and press the Juliao point.

4. Pressing and Kneading the Huantiao Point

Location: In the depression on the outer side of the gluteus maximus, on both sides when standing.

Method: Lie on your side (with the lower leg stretched and upper leg bent) or on the back. Use the thumb or middle finger to press and knead the point forcefully, 20 to 30 times, until some tingling and distension are felt or a feeling of electric shock is radiated to the lower limbs.

Effect: Cure and prevent sciatica, paralysis of the lower limbs, inflammation of the hip, and sprain of surrounding soft tissues.

5. Plucking the Chengfu Point

Location: At the center of the gluteal fold, where the buttock meets the upper leg.

Method: While standing, use the index, middle and ring finger to press the Chengfu point, plucking it from inward to outward for two minutes, until tingling and distension are felt as the best effect.

Effect: Cure waist and buttock pain, sciatica, drooping buttocks, underdeveloped muscle of the buttocks and hemorrhoids.

6. Pressing and Kneading the Yinmen Point

Location: 1.5 cun above the middle point between the gluteal fold and popliteal crease.

Method: Stand with legs spread slightly. Use the middle finger to press the Yinmen point for about one minute. Then continue to press and knead for about another two minutes, until some tingling and distension are felt, radiating upward and downward as the best effect.

Effect: Promote blood circulation, eliminate swelling, tone buttocks and legs while reducing fat accumulation in the thighs, and treat waist-back pain, lower limb paralysis and numbness.

7. Pressing and Kneading the Weiyang Point

Location: With the knee bent, it is above the popliteal transverse line.

Method: Sit with one leg stretched out straight and the other bent slightly. Lean the whole body toward the straight leg with the arm on that side supporting the body. Use one hand to press and knead the Weiyang point clockwise for about two minutes, until tingling and pain are felt as the best effect.

Effect: Cure abdominal distension, difficult urination, severe pain in the lumbar spine, and leg-foot pain with spasm.

8. Pressing and Kneading the Weizhong Point

Location: Right in the middle of popliteal crease (at the back of the knee).

Method: Sit upright. Use the middle or index finger to press the Weizhong point of the affected side, keeping the thumb pressing just outside the patella. Proceed from light to heavy force, repeating 20 to 40 times.

Effect: Cure all kinds of waist-back pain, tingling in the waist, pain and swelling in the legs, pain around the knee joints, and paralysis of the lower limbs. It also eases fatigue all over the body.

9. Pressing the Chengshan Point

Location: In a cavity in the middle of the rear of the lower leg, at the top of the depression between the two muscles of the calf.

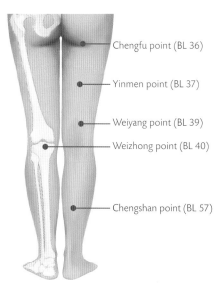

Location of the Chengfu, Yinmen, Weiyang, Weizhong and Chengshan points.

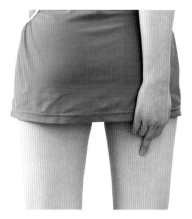

Press and knead the Yinmen point.

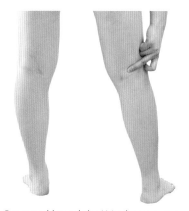

Press and knead the Weizhong point.

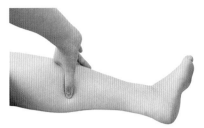

Press the Chengshan point.

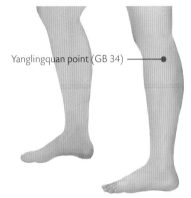

Yanglingquan point (GB 34)

Location of the Yanglingquan point.

Method: Sit upright. Use the thumb to press the Chengshan point for one minute, until some tingling and distension are felt as the best effect.

Effect: Treat waist-back pain, sciatica, spasm of the gastrocnemius muscle in the calf, leg paralysis, thickening in the lower leg, and constipation.

10. Pressing and Kneading the Yanglingquan Point

Location: On the outer side of the shin in a notch at the front lower part of the fibula.

Method: Sit upright. Use the thumb tip to press the Yanglingquan point of the affected side, while putting the other four fingers at the rear of the lower leg, pressing and kneading outward for two to three minutes with slightly heavy force until some tingling and distension are obviously felt. Some patients will feel radiative numbness toward the outer side of the calf.

Effect: Treat jaundice, rib pain, bitter taste in the mouth, vomiting and acid regurgitation from liver and gallbladder problems related to gastric diseases, knee swelling and pain, lower limb paralysis and numbness, knee joint problems and febrile convulsion.

11. Pressing and Kneading the Kunlun Point

Location: In a cavity directly in the rear of the lateral malleolus.

Method: Kneel on one leg. Use the middle finger to press the point vertically for about two minutes.

Effect: Treat ankle sprain, swelling and pain, high blood pressure, insomnia, forgetfulness, menstrual disorder, nocturnal emission, impotence, pain during sexual intercourse, and frequent urination.

Tips
- Avoid catching a cold.
- Be mindful of keeping the waist and affected limb dry after exercise, such as by changing sweaty clothes in timely matter and prevent wet clothes from drying on the body.
- Do not take a bath immediately after sweating.
- Undertake moderate physical exercise for the waist and legs.

18 | Abdominal Pain and Distension

Abdominal pain refers to pain below the stomach and above the symphysis pubis.

Abdominal distension refers to swelling or discomfort in the abdomen, which is a common symptom of digestive system problems. The main reason is flatulence in the gastric system and intestines, as well as ascites and abdominal tumors caused by various reasons.

Symptoms

The patient feels distended and heavy in the abdomen while suffering from belching, fullness, nausea, vomiting, appetite loss and borborygmus. Some patients also suffer from abdominal pain.

Target Acupoints

Shoulder, back and waist: Pishu (BL 20), Weishu (BL 21).
Chest and abdomen: Zhongwan (RN 12), Xiawan (RN 10), Tianshu (ST 25), Shenque (RN 8), Qihai (RN 6), Guanyuan (RN 4).
Arms: Quchi (LI 11), Hegu (LI 4).
Legs: Zusanli (ST 36), Shangjuxu (ST 37), Liangqiu (ST 34), Xiangu (ST 43).

Recommended Massage

1. Pressing and Kneading the Pishu Point
Location: At the point 1.5 cun away horizontally from the eleventh thoracic vertebra.

Method: Sit or stand. Use both middle fingers to press the Pishu point, with the thumb against the ribs, forcefully pressing and kneading for two minutes. Or with a clenched fist, use the index knuckle to press and knead the Pishu point for two minutes. Alternatively you may use a hollow fist to knead and rub it for two minutes, until some tingling and distension are felt.

Effect: Cure nausea, vomiting, abdominal distension, diarrhea, hemafecia (bloody stool) and jaundice.

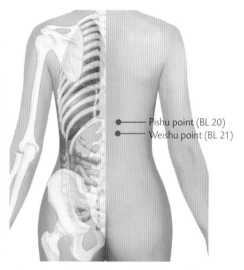

Pishu point (BL 20)
Weishu point (BL 21)

Location of the Pishu and Weishu points.

2. Pressing and Kneading the Weishu Point
Location: About 1.5 cun below the spinous process of the twelfth thoracic vertebra.

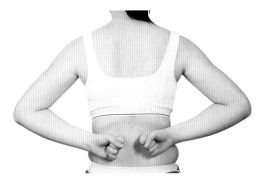

Press and knead the Weishu point.

Method: With a clenched fist, use the knuckle of the index finger to press and knead the Weishu point for two minutes. Or use a hollow fist to knead and rub it for two minutes, until some tingling and distension are felt.

Effect: Treat such diseases of the digestive system as acute or chronic gastritis, gastroptosis, stomach atony, abdominal distension and pain, lack of appetite, nausea and vomiting.

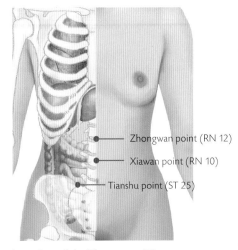

Location of the Zhongwan, Xiawan and Tianshu points.

Zhongwan point (RN 12)

Xiawan point (RN 10)

Tianshu point (ST 25)

3. Pressing and Kneading the Zhongwan Point

Location: In between the lower part of the sternum and the navel.

Method: Lie on the back or sit upright. First use the index or middle finger to press the point for 30 seconds. Then continue to press and knead it for two minutes, until some tingling and distension are felt.

Effect: Treat diseases of the digestive system, such as abdominal distension and pain, diarrhea, nausea and constipation, as well as lack of appetite, dizziness, tinnitus, acne and neurasthenia.

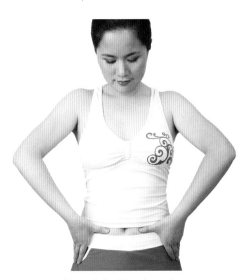

Press and knead the Tianshu point.

4. Pressing and Kneading the Tianshu Point

Location: About two cun horizontally away from the navel.

Method: Lie on the back or sit upright. Use both thumbs or middle fingers to press the Tianshu point on both sides for 30 seconds. Then continue to press and knead for another two minutes, until some tingling and distension are felt, radiating to the entire abdomen as the best effect.

Effect: Cure abdominal distension and pain, nausea, vomiting, constipation, diarrhea, menstrual disorder and dysmenorrhea.

5. Pressing and Kneading the Xiawan Point

Location: Two cun above the navel.

Method: Lie on the back or sit upright. First use the index or middle finger to press the point for 30 seconds. Then continue to press and knead it for another two minutes, until some tingling and distension are felt.

Effect: Cure abdominal distension and pain, diarrhea, acid reflux, vomiting and constipation.

6. Massaging the Shenque Point

Location: At the center of the navel.

Method: Use the right palm to massage around the navel gently and slowly, for two to three minutes in a revolving manner, until warmth is felt in the abdomen. It is better to do it one hour after eating.

Effect: Cure cold and pain around the navel, dysmenorrhea, infertility, cold limbs, diarrhea or constipation, and aconuresis (urinary incontinence).

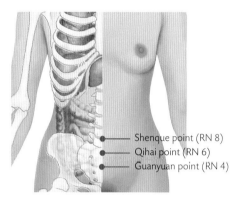

Shenque point (RN 8)
Qihai point (RN 6)
Guanyuan point (RN 4)

Location of the Shenque, Qihai and Guanyuan points.

7. Pressing and Kneading the Qihai Point

Location: About 1.5 cun below the navel.

Method: Use the tips of the index and middle finger to press and knead the point for two minutes, until warmth is felt as the best effect.

Effect: Cure abdominal pain and distension, constipation or diarrhea, menstrual disorder, dysmenorrhea, amenorrhea, impotence, premature ejaculation and nocturnal emission.

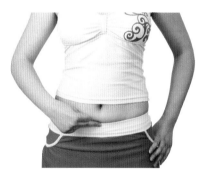

Press and knead the Qihai point.

8. Pressing and Kneading the Guanyuan Point

Location: About three cun below the navel.

Method: Use two palms to press and knead the point for three minutes, until warmth is felt in the abdomen.

Effect: Cure abdominal pain and distension, menstrual disorder, dysmenorrhea, amenorrhea, nocturnal emission and impotence.

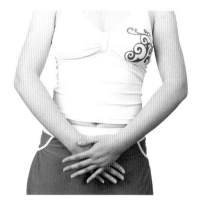

Press and knead the Guanyuan point.

9. Pressing and Kneading the Quchi Point

Location: With the elbow bent halfway, on the outer side of the cubital transverse crease.

Method: Use the thumb pad to press and knead the point for two minutes.

Effect: Ease diarrhea, nasal allergy, headache and elbow joint pain.

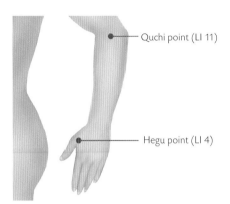
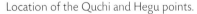

Location of the Quchi and Hegu points.

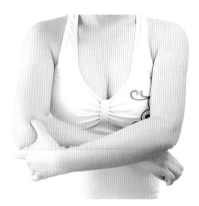

Press and knead the Quchi point.

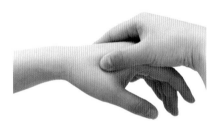

Press and knead the Hegu point.

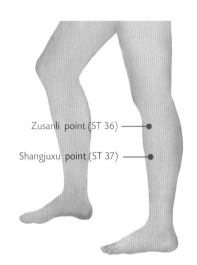

Location of the Zusanli and Shangjuxu points.

10. Pressing and Kneading the Hegu Point

Location: In the highest point on the back of the hand between the thumb base and the base of the index finger (in the webbing between these two fingers).

Method: Use the thumb heel to press the point for three minutes until some tingling and distension are felt as the best effect.

Effect: Cure cold, runny nose, headache, toothache, acne, visual fatigue, sore throat, tinnitus and hiccups.

11. Pressing and Kneading the Zusanli Point

Location: About three cun below the knee on the outer side of the tibia.

Method: Sit upright. Use both thumbs to press the point on both sides, with the four fingers alongside the outer side of the lower leg, pressing and kneading outward 20 to 40 times, until some tingling and distension are felt as the best effect.

Effect: Treat diarrhea, abdominal pain and distension, lack of appetite, constipation, hiccups, vomiting, anemia, low blood pressure, menopause syndrome and waist-leg pain.

12. Pressing the Shangjuxu Point

Location: One middle finger cun (the length of the second section of the middle finger) on the outside of the tibial crest. Three cun below the Zusanli point.

Method: Sit upright. Use both thumbs to press the point, until some tingling and distension are felt as the best effect.

Effect: Treat diseases of the digestive system, such gastric and intestinal inflammation, diarrhea, dysentery, hernia, constipation, indigestion, aftereffect of cerebrovascular diseases, lower-limb paralysis or spasm, and knee swelling with pain.

13. Pressing the Liangqiu Point

Location: With the knee bent, on the outer edge of the thigh, two cun above the outer upper margin of the patella.

Method: Use the thumb to press the point, with the four fingers gripping the thigh from below.

Effect: Control and ease acute gastric symptoms and adjust the digestive system, as well as benefiting foot and knee tingling with pain.

14. Pressing the Xiangu Point

Location: In a cavity before the junction of the second metatarsal and third metatarsal bones.

Method: Sit cross-legged with one knee held up. Use the index finger to press the point for two minutes.

Effect: Cure abdominal pain and distension, borborygmus, diarrhea, facial edema, red eye with pain, hernia, and swelling and pain of the foot dorsum.

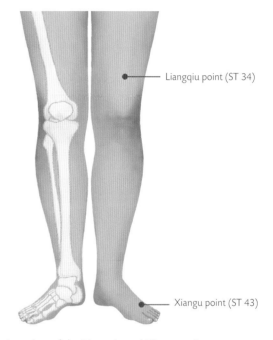

Liangqiu point (ST 34)

Xiangu point (ST 43)

Location of the Liangqiu and Xiangu points.

Tips
- Abdominal pain and abdominal distension after vomiting may be the signal of gastroenteritis, food poisoning or acute gastritis. It is best to have a doctor assess the condition in a timely manner.
- Vomiting after abdominal pain may signal acute appendicitis, pancreatitis and cholecystitis, which require immediate attention at a hospital.
- If there are also symptoms such as hemafecia and fever along with abdominal pain and distension, timely treatment is the key.

19 Intercostal Nerve Pain

It is pain attacking one intercostal region or several intercostal regions along the area distributed with costal nerves, together with severe spasms. It is mostly caused by viral infection, toxin irritation, mechanical injury and external pressure. Primary intercostal nerve pain is very rare.

Symptoms
The pain is mostly marked by prickling or burning along the area of the intercostal nerves. When it attacks, the pain usually radiates from the rear to the front along corresponding intercostal gaps in a semi-circular form. Coughing, deep breaths or sneezing can make it more painful. The pain mostly attacks on one side.

Target Acupoints
Shoulder, back and waist: Ganshu (BL 18), Geshu (BL 17), Danshu (BL 19).
Chest and abdomen: Qimen (LV 14), Riyue (GB 24).
Legs: Qiuxu (GB 40), Yanglingquan (GB 34).

Recommended Massage
1. Pressing and Kneading the Ganshu Point
Location: 1.5 cun away from the ninth thoracic spinal process on the inner side of the scapula.

Method: Sit upright. Use the knuckles of the four fingers to knead the Ganshu point for about two minutes until tingling and distension are felt.

Effect: Treat distension and pain of both sides of the chest, breast pain with swelling, waist-back pain, agitation, irritability, indigestion and aversion to food, neurasthenia, hepatitis, jaundice (icterus), nausea, vomiting, lack of appetite and dizziness.

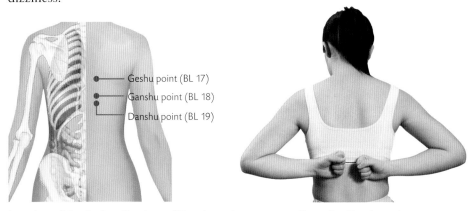

Geshu point (BL 17)
Ganshu point (BL 18)
Danshu point (BL 19)

Location of the Geshu, Ganshu and Danshu points.   Press the Ganshu point.

2. Pressing the Geshu Point

Location: At the point 1.5 cun away from the spinous process of the seventh thoracic vertebra.

Method: Sit on a chair with fists clenched and turned toward the back. Direct the knuckles toward the Geshu point, pressing backward using the body weight.

Effect: Serve to clear the lungs, stop vomiting, promote the circulation of blood and vital energy, and to treat back pain due to blood congestion, sprain of the back muscle, chronic bleeding diseases, prolonged lochiorrhea after giving birth, dizziness resulting from low blood pressure, anemia, hiccups, nervous vomiting, hives and skin diseases.

3. Pressing and Kneading the Danshu Point

Location: At the point 1.5 cun away from the spinous process of the tenth thoracic vertebra.

Method: Sit upright or lie on the back. With fists clenched, use the four knuckles to press and knead the point for about two minutes, until some tingling and distension are felt as the best effect.

Effect: Beneficial for cholecystitis, hepatitis, gastritis, ulcer, vomiting, esophagostenosis, intercostal nerve pain, insomnia, hysteria, gallstones, ascariasis of the biliary tract, pleurisy and high blood pressure.

4. Pressing and Kneading the Qimen Point

Location: In the sixth intercostal space directly below the nipple.

Method: Sit upright or lie on the back. Use the pad of the middle finger to press and knead the Qimen point for two minutes with moderate force, until some tingling, distension and slight warmth are felt as the best effect.

Effect: Cure menstrual disorder, endometritis, abdominal pain, diarrhea, nausea, vomiting, liver pain, cholecystalgia and fatty liver disease.

5. Pressing and Kneading the Riyue Point

Location: In the seventh intercostal space directly below the nipple.

Method: Sit upright or lie on the back. Use the pad of the thumb to press and knead the Riyue point for two minutes, with the four fingers placed on ribs with moderate force, until some tingling, distension and slight warmth are felt as the best effect.

Effect: Treat cholecystitis, gallstones, biliary ascarids, hepatitis, gastric and duodenal ulcer, intercostal nerve pain, phrenospasm and shingles.

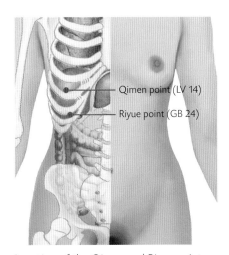

Location of the Qimen and Riyue points.

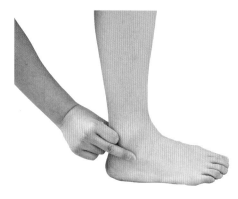

Press and knead the Qiuxu point.

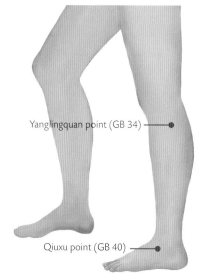

Yanglingquan point (GB 34)

Qiuxu point (GB 40)

Location of the Yanglingquan and Qiuxu points.

6. Pressing and Kneading the Qiuxu Point
Location: In a cavity on the outer side of the extensor tendon.

Method: While squatting use the middle finger to press and knead the Qiuxu point of the affected side outward for two minutes with the thumb attached to the rear of the inner ankle until you cannot bear the force exerted.

Effect: Prevent and cure chest pain, cholecystitis, sciatica, lower-limb paralysis and diseases of the surrounding soft tissues.

7. Pinching the Yanglingquan Point
Location: On the outer side of the shin in a notch at the front lower part of the fibula.

Method: Sit upright. Use the thumb tip to pinch the Yanglingquan point forcefully, with pressure directed toward the toes for about one minute, until obvious tingling and distension are felt as the best effect.

Effect: Treat a variety of ailments, including knee arthritis, diseases of the surrounding soft tissues, lower-limb paralysis, ankle sprain, shoulder periarthritis, stiff neck, pain after intramuscular injection in the hip, lumbar sprain, gallstones, cholecystalgia, ascariasis of the biliary tract, habitual constipation, high blood pressure and intercostal nerve pain.

Tips
- You must pay attention to ascertaining the specific cause of the symptom. Its early stage is very similar to that of shingles, hence requiring careful identification.
- Illness in the thoracic vertebrae should be treated in time to prevent secondary intercostal nerve pain.
- Those always in a seated position at work should be mindful of their posture to prevent fatigue.

20 | Chronic Diarrhea

This describes a condition when defecating frequency obviously exceeds normal, in addition to thin or watery stool, or stool that contains undigested food or mucus and/or blood. It is a common symptom often accompanied by the urgent need to defecate, discomfort of the anus, and incontinence.

Symptoms

There are two kinds of diarrhea, acute and chronic, along with different symptoms.

Acute diarrhea: Thin excrement is discharged more than three times a day, or the amount exceeds 200 grams in which 80 percent is water. The course of diarrhea is within one to two weeks. There are many causes for acute diarrhea. Eating tainted food is a common one.

Chronic diarrhea: Defecating frequency increases, with thin excrement and even mucopurulent bloody stool, lasting for over two months.

Chronic diarrhea caused by pathological changes in the small intestine is marked by abdominal discomfort that becomes more painful after eating or before defecation, along with a large amount of excrement of light color. Defecating frequency varies.

Chronic diarrhea caused by pathological changes in the colon is marked by discomfort in both sides of the abdomen or lower abdomen. The symptoms often diminish after excrement discharge, of a large amount and urgent need, with a small amount often containing blood and mucus.

Chronic diarrhea caused by pathological changes in the rectum is often marked by urgent defecation followed by more serious phenomena: abdominal pain, feeling a constant need to defecate, heaviness of the anus, and discomfort in the course of defecation.

Target Acupoints

Shoulder, back and waist: Pishu (BL 20), Shenshu (BL 23), Baliao(BL 31–34), Dachangshu (BL 25).
Chest and abdomen: Zhongwan (RN 12), Tianshu (ST 25), Qihai (RN 6), Guanyuan (RN 4).
Legs: Zusanli (ST 36), Liangqiu (ST 34).

Recommended Massage

1. Pressing and Kneading the Pishu Point
Location: At the point 1.5 cun away horizontally from the eleventh thoracic vertebra.

Method: Sit or stand. Use both middle fingers to press the Pishu point, with

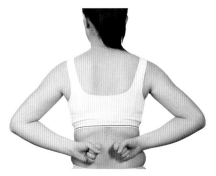

Press and knead the Pishu point.

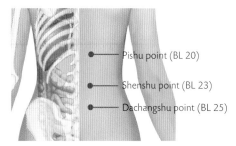

Pishu point (BL 20)

Shenshu point (BL 23)

Dachangshu point (BL 25)

Location of the Pishu, Shenshu and Dachangshu points.

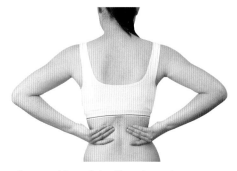

Press and knead the Shenshu point.

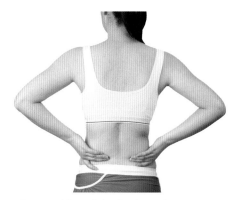

Press and knead the Dachangshu point.

the thumb against the ribs, forcefully pressing and kneading for two minutes. Or with a clenched fist, use the index knuckle to press and knead the Pishu point for two minutes. Alternatively you may use a hollow fist to knead and rub it for two minutes, until some tingling and distension are felt.

Effect: Cure nausea, vomiting, abdominal distension, diarrhea, hemafecia (bloody stool) and jaundice.

2. Pressing and Kneading the Shenshu Point

Location: 1.5 cun horizontally from the second lumbar spinal process.

Method: Lie on the back or sit upright. Use the two middle fingers to forcefully press and knead the Shenshu point of both sides 30 to 50 times, keeping the thumbs by the ribs. Or, with a clenched fist, use the knuckle of the index finger to press and knead the Shenshu point 30 to 50 times. You might also try using a loose fist to knead and rub 30 to 50 times, until some warmth is felt as the best effect.

Effect: Treat waist tingling and leg pain, lumbar muscle strain, lumbar disc herniation, leg swelling, fatigue all over the body, impotence, nocturnal emission, premature ejaculation and menstrual disorder.

3. Pressing and Kneading the Dachangshu Point

Location: About 1.5 cun away from the fourth lumbar vertebra on two sides.

Method: Sit upright or lie on the back. Use the pads of both middle fingers to press and knead the Dachangshu point on each side.

Effect: Treat constipation, abdominal pain, abdominal distension, diarrhea, borborygmus, waist-back pain and premature ejaculation.

4. Kneading and Rubbing the Baliao Points

Location: There are eight Baliao points in total, four on each side of the sacral spine. These are the upper, secondary, middle and lower Baliao points. They are located respectively in the first, second, third and fourth posterior sacral foramina (opening between vertebrae).

    Method: Sit upright. Use the palm to knead, or rub up and down, along the sacral vertebrae for about two minutes, until some tingling and distension are felt as the best effect.

    Effect: Cure pain in the lumbosacral spine, constipation, distension and pain in the lower abdomen, pelvic inflammation, difficult urination, menstrual disorder and hemorrhoids.

5. Pressing and Kneading the Zhongwan Point

Location: In between the lower part of the sternum and the navel.

    Method: Sit upright or lie on the back. Use the middle or index finger to press and knead the point for about two minutes, until some tingling and distension are felt as the best effect.

    Effect: Treat diseases of the digestive system, such as abdominal distension and pain, diarrhea, nausea and constipation, as well as lack of appetite, dizziness, tinnitus, acne and neurasthenia.

6. Pressing and Kneading the Tianshu Point

Location: About two cun horizontally away from the navel.

    Method: Sit upright or lie on the back. Use two thumbs to press and knead the Tianshu point on both sides for several minutes, with the rest of four fingers attached on both sides, until some tingling and distension are felt, ideally radiating to the entire abdomen.

    Effect: Cure abdominal distension and pain, nausea, vomiting, constipation, diarrhea, menstrual disorder and dysmenorrhea.

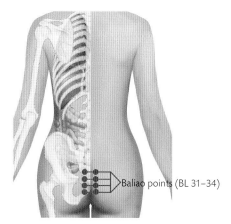

Location of the Baliao points.

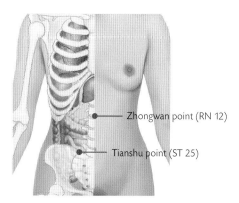

Location of the Zhongwan and Tianshu points.

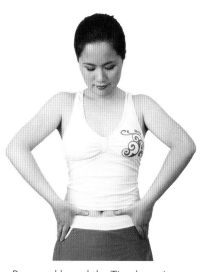

Press and knead the Tianshu point.

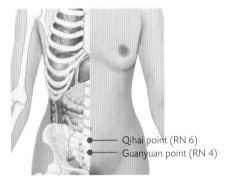

Location of the Qihai and Guanyuan points.

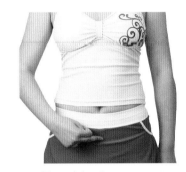

Press and knead the Guanyuan point

7. Pressing and Kneading the Qihai Point

Location: About 1.5 cun below the navel.

Method: Use the tip of the middle finger to press and knead for two minutes, until warmth is felt as the best effect.

Effect: Cure abdominal pain and distension, constipation or diarrhea, menstrual disorder, dysmenorrhea, amenorrhea, impotence, premature ejaculation and nocturnal emission.

8. Pressing and Kneading the Guanyuan Point

Location: About three cun below the navel.

Method: Use the tip of the middle finger to press and knead for two minutes, until warmth is felt as the best effect.

Effect: Cure abdominal pain and distension, menstrual disorder, dysmenorrhea, amenorrhea, nocturnal emission and impotence.

9. Pressing and Kneading the Zusanli Point

Location: About three cun below the knee on the outer side of the tibia.

Method: Sit upright. Use both thumbs to press the point on both sides, with the four fingers alongside the outer side of the lower leg, pressing and kneading outward 20 to 40 times, until some tingling and distension are felt as the best effect.

Effect: Treat diarrhea, abdominal pain and distension, lack of appetite, constipation, hiccups, vomiting, anemia, low blood pressure, menopause syndrome and waist-leg pain.

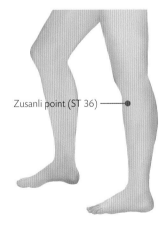
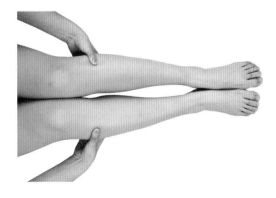

Press and knead the Zusanli point.

10. Pressing the Liangqiu Point

Location: With the knee bent, on the outer edge of the thigh, two cun above the outer upper margin of the patella.

Method: Sit upright. Use two thumbs to press and knead the point, with the body leaning toward the Liangqiu point being massaged.

Effect: Cure gastric convulsion, mastitis, knee-joint pain and acute gastricpain.

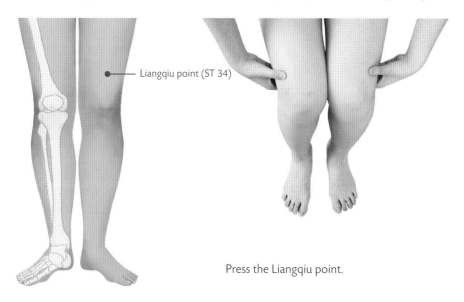

Liangqiu point (ST 34)

Press the Liangqiu point.

Tips

The causes of chronic diarrhea are quite complex, since it is not necessarily caused by intestinal inflammation, hence requiring careful and serious examination.

- Diabetes: Diarrhea caused by diabetes is stubborn and continual, lasting for several days or weeks, and can reoccur any time within weeks or months in the daytime or at night. This is related to pathological changes of the autonomic nerves in the gastric and intestinal tracts caused by diabetes.
- Hyperthyroidism: These cases are marked by quick movement of the intestinal tract, undesirable digestion and absorption, and frequent defecation and even diarrhea. The excrement generally appears mushy, containing much undigested food.
- Colorectal cancer: This happens mostly after middle age. When the cancer is marked by erosion, ulcer and necrosis, there may be diarrhea, bloody stool and feeling an urgent need to defecate.

21 | Lateral Femoral Cutaneous Neuritis

The patient feels that the area encompassing two-thirds of the outer frontal part of the lower thigh is cold, numb, painful and even burning. It happens mostly on one side. Some patients have more serious symptoms after standing up, walking or catching a cold. This illness is mostly caused by lumbar injury or compression of skin nerves in the outer flank of the thigh.

Symptoms

It often happens to middle-aged males, with gradual progression. At the beginning the pain is frequent, gradually becoming continuous and sometimes very severe. Friction of clothes, forceful movements, standing up or walking for a long time can all make it worse. Medical examination shows that normal feeling, pain sensation and the ability to feel temperature on the skin of the frontal outer thigh diminish or even disappear. Some patients also suffer from skin atrophy, however without muscle atrophy. The tendon reflection exists normally without restriction of movement.

Target Acupoints

Legs: Fengshi (GB 31), Futu (ST 32), Yanglingquan (GB 34), Liangqiu (ST 34).

Recommended Massage

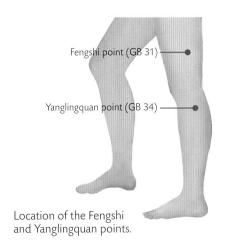

Fengshi point (GB 31)

Yanglingquan point (GB 34)

Location of the Fengshi and Yanglingquan points.

1. Pressing the Fengshi Point

Location: With the arm lying naturally at the side, the point where the tip of the middle finger touches the leg.

Method: Stand straight or lie down on the side. Use the tip of the middle finger to press the point 20 to 30 times. You can also sit upright and use the thumb to press the point 20 to 30 times, until some tingling and distension are felt as the best effect.

Effect: Cure tingling and pain in the leg, paralysis, pain in the waist, sciatica, skin itch and hives.

2. Pinching the Yanglingquan Point

Location: On the outer side of the shin in a notch at the front lower part of the fibula.

Method: Sit upright. Use the thumb tip to pinch the Yanglingquan point forcefully, with pressure directed toward the toes for about one minute, until obvious tingling and distension are felt as the best effect.

Effect: Treat jaundice, rib pain, bitter taste in the mouth, vomiting and acid regurgitation from liver and gallbladder problems related to gastric diseases, knee swelling and pain, lower limb paralysis and numbness, knee joint problems and febrile convulsion.

3. Pressing and Kneading the Futu Point

Location: Six cun above the outer upper margin of the patella.

Method: Sit upright. Use the thumb pad to press the Futu point of the affected side for two minutes, until some tingling and distension are felt as the best effect.

Effect: Cure paralysis of the lower limbs, waist pain, coldness in the knee, hernia and dermatophytosis.

4. Pressing and Kneading the Liangqiu Point

Location: With the knee bent, on the outer edge of the thigh, two cun above the outer upper margin of the patella.

Method: Sit upright. Use the thumb tip to press and knead the Liangqiu point of the affected side for two minutes, until some tingling and distension are felt as the best effect.

Effect: Treat diseases of the digestive system such as gastric convulsion, gastritis, diarrhea and vomiting; diseases of gynecology and obstetrics such as mastitis and dysmenorrhea; and orthopedic issues such as rheumatic arthritis, suprapatellar bursitis, chondromalacia patellae and pathological changes in the knee joints.

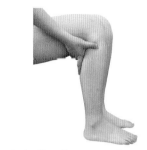

Pinch the Yanglingquan point.

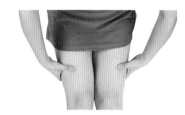

Press and knead the Futu point.

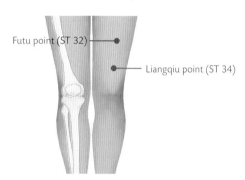

Futu point (ST 32)

Liangqiu point (ST 34)

Location of the Futu and Liangqiu points.

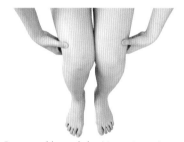

Press and knead the Liangqiu point.

Tips
- Acupuncture and moxibustion therapy have quite beneficial effects.
- Be mindful of keeping the affected part warm.

22 | Tennis Elbow

Also called external humeral epicondylitis, it is generally caused by excessive pulling and stretching of muscles due to revolution, bending and extension of the forearm through excessive force. As might be expected from the name, playing tennis over a long time may lead to this illness.

Symptoms

In most patients this develops slowly. At the beginning patients only feel tingling and slight pain in the outside of the elbow. They cannot hold things tightly. Actions such as lifting pots, twisting towels and knitting sweaters will make it worse. Those with serious cases will suffer from pain when stretching the fingers and wrists or holding utensils.

Pain in the affected limb will be eased with a relaxed state of the extensor muscle group as the limb is bent and the forearm revolved backward. A few patients will feel more pain on overcast or rainy days.

Target Acupoints

Arms: Jianzhen (SI 9), Quze (PC 3), Quchi (LI 11) and Shousanli (LI 10).

Recommended Massage

1. Pressing and Kneading the Jianzhen Point
Location: At the lower back of the shoulder joint.

Method: Use the middle finger to press, rub and knead the Jianzhen point for two minutes with moderate force until you feel obviously tingling and distension in the part concerned.

Effect: Cure problems with the joints and soft tissues of the shoulder as well as upper limb paralysis and armpit sweating.

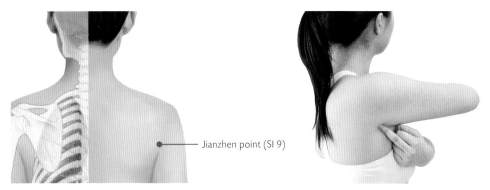

Jianzhen point (SI 9)

Press and knead the Jianzhen point.

2. Pressing the Quze Point

Location: With the elbow bent slightly, within the inner lateral margin of the biceps brachii on the cubital crease.

Method: Sit upright. Use the middle finger to press the point with the bone-joint close to the bent thumb in order to exert force.

Effect: Treat heart pain, palpitation, problems resulting from heat, agitation, gastric pain, vomiting, elbow-arm pain, arm trembling, rheumatic heart disease, chorea minor, acute gastric and intestinal diseases, bronchitis and heat-stroke.

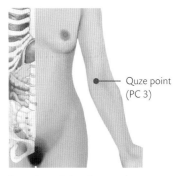

Quze point (PC 3)

Location of the Quze point.

3. Pinching and Kneading the Quchi Point

Location: With the elbow bent halfway, on the outer side of the cubital transverse crease.

Method: Sit upright with the arm bent halfway. Use the thumb of the other hand to pinch and press the Quchi point for one minute. Then press and knead for another two minutes, until some tingling and distension are felt.

Effect: Cure arm swelling, weakness in the hands and elbow, and arm paralysis.

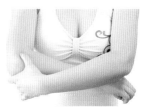

Pinch and knead the Quchi point.

4.Pressing and Kneading the Shousanli Point

Location: Two cun below the Quchi point.

Method: With forearm bent slightly, use the thumb pad to press and knead the point for two minutes, proceeding from light to heavy force, until some tingling and distension are felt as the best effect.

Effect: Treat arm paralysis, periarthritis, upper-limb neuralgia, lumbar pain, gastroptosis, ulcer, acute and chronic enteritis, indigestion, toothache, oral ulcer, cervical adenitis, facioplegia, facial convulsion, mastitis and cold.

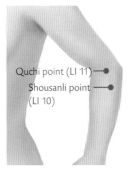

Quchi point (LI 11)

Shousanli point (LI 10)

Location of the Quchi and Shousanli points.

Tips

As the pain of tennis elbow attacks repeatedly, it is advisable to persist in the combination of prevention and treatment, with stress on the former, and try to avoid or reduce movements detrimental to recovery.

- When playing tennis and badminton, choose a light and elastic racket of high quality to reduce the burden of the arm.
- Try not to lift heavy things.
- Be mindful of the wrist position during actions such as lifting a pot, pouring water and wringing clothes. When mopping, bend legs slightly and use the force of the waist and legs rather than only using the arm.
- Try as much as possible to reduce the amount of work when the symptoms are present, in order to prevent the condition from becoming worse.

23 | Arm Pain

This is common among manual laborers. Also when cooking and washing clothes or dishes, housewives may feel fatigue in the arm, hence making it easy for them to contract chronic inflammation. Arm pain often happens along with tennis elbow and inflammation of styloid process.

Symptoms

Arm pain often attacks in the area where the bone can be felt slightly upward of the elbow and in the plumpest part of the forearm muscle. Very often the patient cannot bend or stretch the wrist joint when the pain attacks, and the pain will be more obvious when the patient twists a towel. A sound may be even heard when the patient moves the arm.

Target Acupoints

Arms: Chize (LU 5), Quchi (LI 11), Yangchi (SJ 4), Shousanli (LI 10), Waiguan (SJ 5), Kongzui (LU 6), Hegu (LI 4).

Recommended Massage

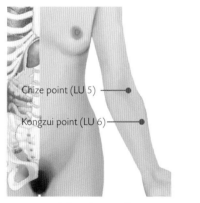

Location of the Chize and Kongzui points.

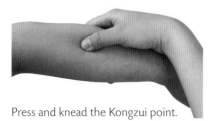

Press and knead the Kongzui point.

1. Pinching and Kneading the Chize Point

Location: With the elbow bent slightly, in a cavity of the outer side of the biceps brachii on the cubital crease.

Method: Sit with the arm bent halfway. Use the thumb tip to pinch and knead the point for one minute and then continue for another two minutes, until some tingling and distension are felt as the best effect.

Effect: Cure arm pain, elbow-joint pain, sore throat, cough, chest pain, heart pain and hematemesis.

2. Pressing and Kneading the Kongzui Point

Location: About seven cun above the wrist crease, with the palm turned upward.

Method: Bend the forearm slightly. Use the thumb pad to press and knead the point for two minutes, proceeding from light to heavy force, until some tingling and distension are felt as the best effect.

Effect: Cure tennis elbow, forearm tingling and pain, hemorrhoids, asthma, cough, hematemesis and sore throat.

3. Pinching and Pressing the Quchi Point

Location: With the elbow bent halfway, on the outer side of the cubital transverse crease.

Method: Sit upright with the arm bent halfway. Use the thumb of the other hand to pinch and press the Quchi point for one minute. Then press and knead for another two minutes, until some tingling and distension are felt.

Effect: Cure arm swelling, weakness in the hands and elbow, and arm paralysis.

4.Pressing and Kneading the Shousanli Point

Location: Two cun below the Quchi point.

Method: With forearm bent slightly, use the thumb pad to press and knead the point for two minutes, proceeding from light to heavy force, until some tingling and distension are felt as the best effect.

Effect: Treat arm paralysis, periarthritis, upper-limb neuralgia, lumbar pain, gastroptosis, ulcer, acute and chronic enteritis, indigestion, toothache, oral ulcer, cervical adenitis, facioplegia, facial convulsion, mastitis and cold.

5. Pressing and Kneading the Yangchi Point

Location: In a cavity of the ulnar margin of the exterior muscles of the fingers.

Method: Bend the forearm halfway. Use the pad of the thumb to forcefully press and knead the Yangchi point of the affected side for three minutes, until some tingling and distension are felt, ideally radiating numbness to the palm and fingers.

Effect: Cure red eyes with swelling and pain, sore throat, and problems with wrist joints and surrounding soft tissues.

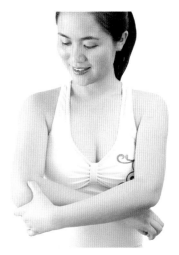

Pinch and knead the Quchi point.

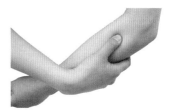

Press and knead the Shousanli point.

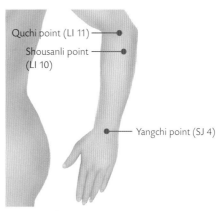

Quchi point (LI 11)

Shousanli point (LI 10)

Yangchi point (SJ 4)

Location of the Quchi, Shousanli and Yangchi points.

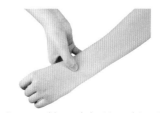

Press and knead the Yangchi point.

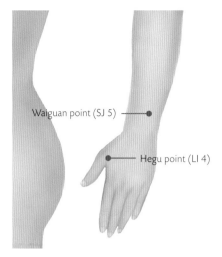

Location of the Waiguan and Hegu points.

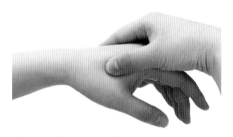

Pinch and knead the Hegu point.

6. Pressing and Kneading the Waiguan Point

Location: In the middle on the outside of the arm, between the ulna and radius about two cun away from the horizontal line of the wrist joint.

Method: With the forearm bent halfway, use the pad of the thumb on the healthy side of the body to forcefully press the Waiguan point of the affected side. Move for three minutes, until some tingling and distension are felt, ideally radiating numbness to the palm and fingers.

Effect: Cure fever, cold, pneumonia, tinnitus, dumbness, stiff neck, migraine, intercostal nerve pain, upper limb joint pain, and elbow pain.

7. Pinching and Kneading the Hegu Point

Location: In the highest point on the back of the hand between the thumb base and the base of the index finger (in the webbing between these two fingers).

Method: Use the thumb to press the Hegu point on the other hand 10 to 20 times alternatively from light to heavy force until tingling and distension are felt as the best effect.

Effect: Treat cold, runny nose, headache, toothache, acne, visual fatigue, sore throat, tinnitus and hiccups.

Tips

Hand, wrist, elbow and arm pain may be caused as follows:

- Bone fracture: With severe pain, there is also the deformation of the arm that is likely caused by the injury of the muscle and ligaments in this part.
- Pyogenic osteomyelitis: Inflammation usually caused by infection, it is most often seen among children. It is accompanied by pain in the finger joints, wrists and elbow, as well as swelling and fever.
- Rheumatoid arthritis: Most often seen among women, it is chiefly associated with pathological changes in hand and foot joints among other places. When it attacks the affected joint is obviously painful with restricted movement.

24 | Carpal Tunnel Syndrome

It refers to when the median nerve is pressed within the carpal tunnel, leading to numbness of three and half fingers on the radialis. This syndrome, which is quite common, is mostly related to white collar work particularly at the computer. There are more female than male patients, mostly female office workers aged from 30 to 50. It attacks more on the right side than on the left side.

Symptoms

Those with this syndrome suffer from gradual hand numbness, burning, wrist joint swelling, inflexibility of hand movement and weakness. The pain becomes severe in the evening, even to the extent of affecting sleep.

Target Acupoints

Arms: Neiguan (PC 6), Daling (PC 7), Yangxi (LI 5), Waiguan (SJ 5), Yangchi (SJ 4).

Recommended Massage

1. Pressing and Kneading the Neiguan Point
Location: Between the two tendons about two cun above the wrist joint bend.

Method: Bend the forearm halfway. Use the pad of the thumb to forcefully press and knead the Neiguan point of the affected side for three minutes, until some tingling and distension are felt as the best effect.

Effect: Treat continuous hiccups, nausea, agitation, anxiety, palpitation, angina pectoris, chest distress, chest pain, coronary heart disease, insomnia, gastric and intestinal neurosis.

2. Pressing and Kneading the Daling Point
Location: In the middle of the lateral band of the palm.

Method: Bend the forearm halfway. Use the pad of the thumb to forcefully press and knead the Daling point of the affected side for three minutes, until some tingling and distension are felt, ideally radiating to the palm and fingers.

Effect: Cure heart pain, continuous laugh, epilepsy, bad breath, excessive saliva, cough, hematemesis, wrist sprain and pain.

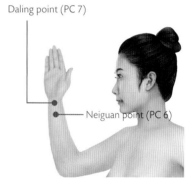

Daling point (PC 7)

Neiguan point (PC 6)

Location of Daling and Neiguan points.

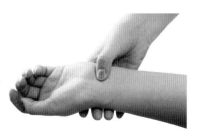

Press and knead the Daling point.

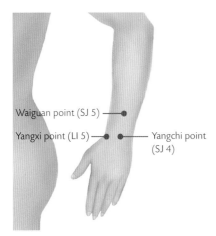

Location of the Waiguan, Yangxi and Yangchi points.

Waiguan point (SJ 5)

Yangxi point (LI 5)

Yangchi point (SJ 4)

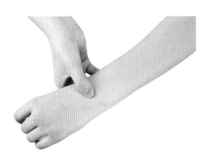

Press and knead the Yangchi point.

3. Pressing and Kneading the Yangxi Point
Location: At the wrist on the thumb side in a notch between two strained tendons when the thumb tilts upward.

Method: With the front arm bent halfway, use one thumb pad to press the Yangxi point of the other hand. Press, rub and knead for two to three minutes until tingling and distension are felt in the part concerned.

Effect: Cure wrist joint pain, peritendinitis, problems with the wrist joints and surrounding soft tissues, front arm pain, paralysis of one side of the body, headache, red and swollen eyes with pain and deafness

4. Pressing and Kneading the Yangchi Point
Location: In a cavity of the ulnar margin of the exterior muscles of the fingers.

Method: Bend the forearm halfway. Use the pad of the thumb to forcefully press and knead the Yangchi point of the affected side for three minutes, until some tingling and distension are felt, ideally radiating numbness to the palm and fingers.

Effect: Cure red eyes with swelling and pain, sore throat, and problems with wrist joints and surrounding soft tissues.

5. Pressing the Waiguan Point
Location: The Waiguan point is in the middle on the outside of the arm, between the ulna and radius about two cun away from the horizontal line of the wrist joint.

Method: With the forearm bent halfway, use the pad of the thumb on the healthy side of the body to forcefully press the Waiguan point of the affected side. Move for three minutes, until some tingling and distension are felt, ideally radiating numbness to the palm and fingers.

Effect: Cure fever, cold, pneumonia, tinnitus, dumbness, stiff neck, migraine, intercostal nerve pain, upper limb joint pain, and elbow pain.

Tips
- Patients in the early stage of this illness should take a full rest. When necessary they should use plaster splints to keep the wrists straight.
- In serious cases surgery is likely. Neglect over a long time may lead to injury of the nerves, darkened palms and atrophied muscles.

25 | Thecal Cyst

Also called wrist cyst, it is often seen on the back of the wrist joints, back of the feet and the armpit. It mostly takes place among young and middle-aged women.

The cyst is caused by the degeneration of connective tissue around the joint capsule. It can be pushed since it is soft in the superficial part of the skin.

Thecal cyst is generally treated through squeezing or tapping to break it, followed by gradual self-absorption. However it may recur. Thecal cysts in some patients can disappear on their own, although it may take quite a long time.

Symptoms

The cyst is mostly attached to the joint capsule or within the tendon sheath. It has colorless, transparent, orange or light yellow thick and sticky liquid inside. There is a small swelling growing slowly outside, appearing round or oval above the skin. At the beginning it is soft and slightly jiggly when touched. Gradually it harden since it has become fibrous.

Most patients do not have any symptoms; only a few feel tingling and pain in the affected part. In rare cases they may feel numb or suffer from muscle paralysis since the nerve of the affected part is pressed by the cyst.

A thecal cyst in the popliteal space may be as big as an egg when the patient stretches the knee. It is hidden in the crease, making it difficult to be found when the patient bends the knee.

Target Acupoints

Arms: Pain point, Yangchi (SJ 4).

Tips
- It is inflammation caused by repeated and excessive friction. Therefore the patient should avoid doing excessive manual labor and keep the affected part under care.
- Make sure that the posture at work is correct to avoid excessive joint strain, while resting regularly.
- Do not use the computer for a long time, resting for five to ten minutes every hour.
- Do more indoor exercise during rest, including stretching or some massage.
- Exercise the muscles at the shoulders, neck, arms and wrists so as to increase elasticity and strengthen muscle force.

Recommended Massage

1. Pressing and Kneading the Pain Point
Location: At the top of the cyst.

Method: Sit upright, with the wrist of the affected side placed flatly on a table and the palm slightly bent. Use the thumb to press and knead the cyst clockwise for five to ten minutes, proceeding from light to heavy force, until you cannot bear the extent of force.

Effect: Channel meridians and collaterals, eliminate inflammation and stop pain.

2. Pressing and Kneading the Yangchi Point
Location: In a cavity of the ulnar margin of the exterior muscles of the fingers.

Method: Bend the forearm halfway. Use the pad of the thumb to forcefully press and knead the Yangchi point of the affected side for three minutes, until some tingling and distension are felt, ideally radiating numbness to the palm and fingers.

Effect: Cure red eyes with swelling and pain, sore throat, and problems with wrist joints and surrounding soft tissues.

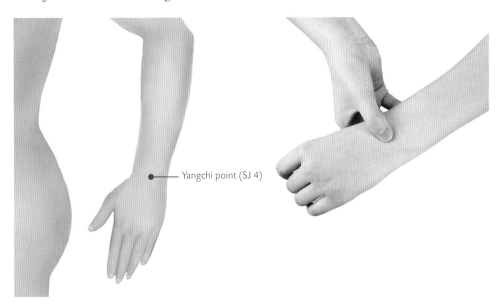

Yangchi point (SJ 4)

Press and knead the Yangchi point.

26 | Wrist Joint Sprain

It refers to an injury of ligaments and tendons around the wrist joints due to external force, leading to internal bleeding or light laceration of tendons and ligaments. Wrist sprain is mostly marked by a history of obvious trauma.

Symptoms

After the sprain there will be weakness of the wrist and inflexibility of the wrist joints. Generally speaking there is no obvious swelling and less pain for those with light sprain, except for pain when the joints move around a lot. For those with severe sprain, there is wrist swelling and greater pain, inability to move the joints or intensified pain during wrist movement.

Target Acupoints

Arms: Yangchi (SJ 4), Yangxi (LI 5), Yanggu (SI 5), Waiguan (SJ 5), Neiguan (PC 6), Daling (PC 7), Wangu (SI 4).

Recommended Massage

1. Pressing and Kneading the Yangchi Point
Location: In a cavity of the ulnar margin of the exterior muscles of the fingers.
    Method: Bend the forearm halfway. Use the pad of the thumb to forcefully press and knead the Yangchi point of the affected side for three minutes, until some tingling and distension are felt, ideally radiating numbness to the palm and fingers.
    Effect: Cure red eyes with swelling and pain, sore throat, and problems with wrist joints and surrounding soft tissues.

2. Pressing and Kneading the Yangxi Point
Location: At the wrist on the thumb side in a notch between two strained tendons when the thumb tilts upward.
    Method: With the front arm bent halfway, use one thumb pad to press the Yangxi point of the other hand. Press, rub and knead for two to three minutes until tingling and distension are felt in the part concerned.
    Effect: Cure wrist joint pain, peritendinitis, problems with the wrist joints and surrounding soft tissues, front arm pain, paralysis of one side of the body, headache, red and swollen eyes with pain and deafness.

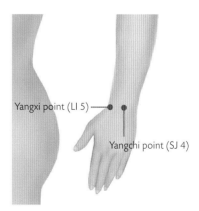

Yangxi point (LI 5)

Yangchi point (SJ 4)

Location of the Yangxi and Yangchi points.

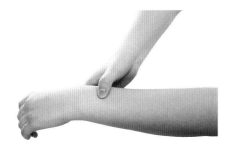

Press the Waiguan point.

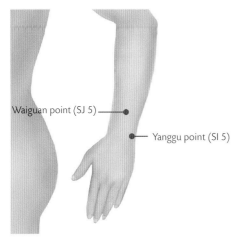

Waiguan point (SJ 5)

Yanggu point (SI 5)

Location of the Waiguan and Yanggu points.

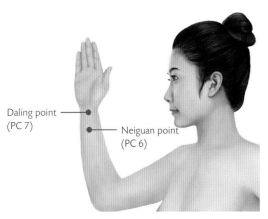

Daling point (PC 7)

Neiguan point (PC 6)

Location of the Daling and Neiguan points.

3. Pressing the Waiguan Point

Location: In the middle on the outside of the arm, between the ulna and radius about two cun away from the horizontal line of the wrist joint.

Method: With the forearm bent halfway, use the pad of the thumb on the healthy side of the body to forcefully press the Waiguan point of the affected side. Move for three minutes, until some tingling and distension are felt, ideally radiating numbness to the palm and fingers.

Effect: Cure fever, cold, pneumonia, tinnitus, dumbness, stiff neck, migraine, intercostal nerve pain, upper limb joint pain, and elbow pain.

4. Pressing and Kneading the Yanggu Point

Location: At the end of the ulnar side of the transverse wrist crease.

Method: Bend the forearm halfway. Use the pad of the thumb to forcefully press and knead the Yanggu point of the affected side for three minutes, until some tingling and distension are felt as the best effect.

Effect: Cure wrist sprain, headache, visual dizziness, tinnitus and deafness.

5. Pressing and Kneading the Daling Point

Location: In the middle of the lateral band of the palm.

Method: Bend the forearm halfway. Use the pad of the thumb to forcefully press and knead the Daling point of the affected side for three minutes, until some tingling and distension are felt, ideally radiating to the palm and fingers.

Effect: Cure heart pain, continuous laugh, epilepsy, bad breath, excessive saliva, cough, hematemesis, wrist sprain and pain.

6. Pressing and Kneading the Neiguan Point

Location: Between the two tendons about two cun above the wrist joint bend.

Method: Bend the forearm halfway. Use the pad of the thumb to forcefully press and knead the Neiguan point of the affected side for three minutes, until some tingling and distension are felt, ideally radiating to the palm and fingers.

Effect: Treat continuous hiccups, nausea, vomiting, agitation, anxiety, palpitation, angina, chest distress or pain, coronary heart disease, insomnia, gastric and intestinal neurosis, wrist sprain and pain.

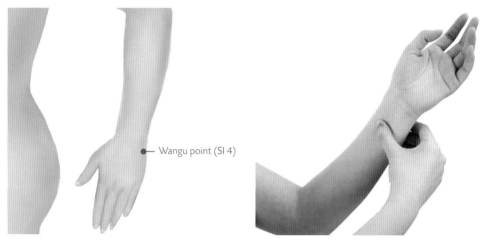

Location of the Wangu point.   Press and knead the Neiguan point.

7. Pressing and Kneading the Wangu Point

Location: In a cavity between the base of the fifth metacarpal bone and the triangle bone.

Method: Use the thumb to press and knead the point for three minutes, proceeding from light to heavy force.

Effect: Treat the absence of sweat with fever, malaria, diabetes, child screaming at night, jaundice, tinnitus, decline of eyesight, tear shedding, headache, neck pain, arm pain and wrist sprain.

Tips

In the early stage of sprain there is red swelling in the affected part. A cold compress with ice cubes or a cold towel can be applied within 24 hours to prevent further swelling. This should be followed by application of hot water to improve blood circulation and promote the absorption of stagnant blood for a better effect.

27 | Knee Pain

Knee joints are complex and heavily used joints of the human body, being apt to result in pathological changes. Common ailments include rheumatic arthritis, meniscus injury and hyperplastic knee arthritis among others.

Symptoms

Symptoms differ since the knee pain can be caused by varied pathological changes.

Rheumatic arthritis is chiefly marked by tingling and pain associated with climatic changes.

Meniscus injury results from trauma, and the patient often feels pain in the points just outside the patella on both sides. Hyperplastic knee arthritis is often found among middle-aged and older people. Increased movement will make the pain severe and the pain will ease after a short rest.

Target Acupoints

Legs: Xiyan (EX-LE 4, ST 35), Weizhong (BL 40), Ququan (LV 8), Xuehai (SP 10), Liangqiu (ST 34), Jiexi (ST 41).

Recommended Massage

1. Pressing and Kneading the Xiyan Points

Location: With the knee bent, in the cavities between the patella and the inner and outer sides of the patellar ligament ("knee eyes").

Method: Sit with knees bent. Use two thumbs to press the inner and outer Xiyan point of the affected side for one minute. Then continue outward for another two minutes, until tingling and distension are felt in the knee joints.

Effect: Cure tingling and distension of knee joints.

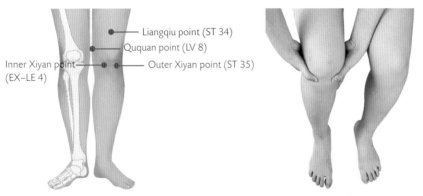

Liangqiu point (ST 34)
Ququan point (LV 8)
Inner Xiyan point (EX–LE 4)
Outer Xiyan point (ST 35)

Location of the Liangqiu, Ququan and Xiyan points.   Press and knead the Xiyan points.

2. Pressing and Kneading the Ququan Point

Location: With the knee bent, in the medial surface of the inner side of the knee.

Method: Sit with the knee bent. Use the index finger to press and knead the point 30 times, proceeding from light to heavy force.

Effect: Cure difficult urination, nocturnal emission, itches in the genital area and knee pain.

3. Pressing and Kneading the Weizhong Point

Location: Right in the middle of popliteal crease (at the back of the knee).

Method: Sit upright. Use the middle or index finger to press the Weizhong point of the affected side, keeping the thumb pressing just outside the patella. Proceed from light to heavy force, repeating 20 to 40 times.

Effect: Cure all kinds of waist-back pain, tingling in the waist, pain and swelling in the legs, pain around the knee joints, and paralysis of the lower limbs. It also eases fatigue all over the body.

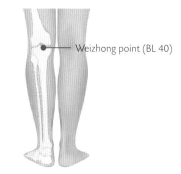

Location of the Weizhong point.

4. Pressing and Kneading the Xuehai Point and the Liangqiu Point

Location: The Xuehai point is in a cavity about two cun away from the inner upper corner of the patella, when the knee is bent. For Liangqiu point, it is in a cavity two cun above the outer upper corner of the patella.

Method: Use one thumb to press the Xuehai point while using the other thumb to press the Liangqiu point at the same time.

Effect: Cure gastric convulsion, mastitis, dizziness and visual dizziness, menstrual disorder, dysmenorrhea, amenorrhea, hives, eczema, coarse skin, skin itch and knee-joint pain.

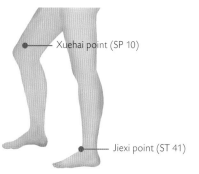

Location of the Xuehai and Jiexi points.

5. Pressing and Kneading the Jiexi Point

Location: In the middle at the front of the ankle.

Method: Sit upright and place the calf on the thigh of the opposite side. Use the thumb to forcefully press and knead the point 20 to 30 times, until tingling and distension are felt as the best effect.

Effect: Prevent and cure ankle sprain, foot arch droop, leg numbness, head-face edema, headache, dizziness, panic, abdominal distension and constipation.

Tips

Inflammation is generally marked by red swelling, heat and pain in the knee. It requires careful diagnosis, so it is better to see a doctor before undertaking targeted treatment.

28 | Calf Muscle Convulsion

This muscle spasm is mostly caused by excessive hard work, putting the ankle in the state of dorsiflexion and the gastrocnemius muscle in a constant state of tension.

Symptoms

Calf muscle convulsion mostly attacks at night, awakening people due to the pain. The pain in the rear of the calf attacks severely and a hard bulge can often be felt.

For some people the symptom can be eased if they exert force to bend the foot back at the time of spasm. For a few people, their sleep will be affected due to the distension of the legs related to frequent movements. People with a severe case may suffer from paralysis of the gastrocnemius muscle.

In addition when swimming, working or undertaking other physical activities, people may also suffer from muscle convulsion with severe pain, restriction over movement, and inability to walk.

Target Acupoints

Legs: Chengjin (BL 56), Weizhong (BL 40), Lougu (SP 7), Chengshan (BL 57).

Recommended Massage

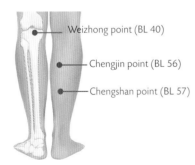

Weizhong point (BL 40)

Chengjin point (BL 56)

Chengshan point (BL 57)

Location of the Weizhong, Chengjin and Chengshan points.

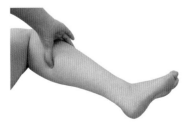

Press and knead the Chengjin point.

1. Pressing and Kneading the Chengjin Point

Location: In the middle of the gastrocnemius muscle; or on the highest prominence of the calf muscle if lying down or sitting upright with the foot slack.

Method: Sitting cross-legged, hold up one knee, fixed by one hand, while using the full surface of the thumb of the other hand to press and knead the Chengjin point in a circular manner. You can also use the thumb to press and knead the Chengjin point of the affected side for two minutes, proceeding from light to heavy force, until tingling and distension are felt as the best effect.

Effect: Chiefly serves to cure waist and leg spasm, pain and hemorrhoids.

2. Pressing and Kneading the Weizhong Point

Location: Right in the middle of popliteal crease (at the back of the knee).

Method: Sit upright. Use the middle or index finger to press the Weizhong point of the affected side, keeping the thumb pressing just outside the patella. Proceed from light to heavy force, repeating 20 to 40 times.

Effect: Cure all kinds of waist-back pain, tingling in the waist, pain and swelling in the legs, pain around the knee joints, and paralysis of the lower limbs. It also eases fatigue all over the body.

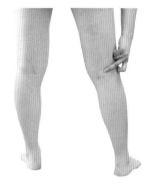

Press and knead the Wezhong point.

3. Pressing the Chengshan Point

Location: Location: In a cavity in the middle of the rear of the lower leg, at the top of the depression between the two muscles of the calf.

Method: Sit upright. Use the thumb to press the Chengshan point of the affected side for two to three minutes generally, proceeding from light to heavy force, until tingling and distension are felt in the rear of the calf as the best effect.

Effect: Chiefly serve to cure calf muscle convulsion, sciatica, waist-back pain, leg paralysis, hemorrhoids, archoptosis and constipation.

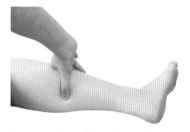

Press and knead the Chengshan point.

4. Pressing and Kneading the Lougu Point

Location: In the rear of the inner lateral margin of the tibia, six cun from the inner ankle tip.

Method: Sit cross-legged with one knee held up and fixed by the hand. Use the finger pad to press and knead the point in a large area for two minutes.

Effect: Chiefly serve to cure acute and chronic intestinal and gastric inflammation, hyperactive bowel sounds, indigestion, scapula pain, leg paralysis, urinary tract infection and mental disorder.

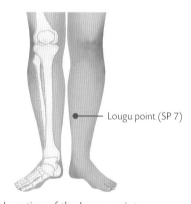

Lougu point (SP 7)

Location of the Lougu point.

Tips

With calf spasm during movement, one should bend the foot back at once, generally lasting for one to two minutes to achieve alleviation effectively. Then massage and knead the calf muscles for 10 minutes to improve blood circulation.

In addition local hot compress can be applied to speed up blood circulation to quickly do away with the spasm.

29 | Ankle Sprain

It is generally caused by training on uneven ground, or excessive pull or laceration of surrounding ligaments due to too much movement of the ankle in a certain direction when one walks downstairs or along a slope. There will be obvious pain in the ankle, restriction over movement and difficulty in walking, even to the extent of avulsion fracture.

This is a common athletic injury, accounting for about 20 to 40 percent of all athletic injuries.

Since the ankle is the hub and a weight-bearing joint, its state has a direct influence on quality of life and capacity for athletic activities.

Symptoms

There can be varied clinical manifestations of ankle sprain related to different injured parts.

Injury of the lateral ligament: It is mostly caused by forceful inward turning (varus) of the foot. In other words, there are pain and swelling in the outer ankle, limping and sometimes stagnant blood under the skin. The lateral ligaments feel painful when pressed, and when the foot turns inward this pain will be more severe. It is rare to see a complete break of the lateral ligaments, but some pain will be more obvious. Due to the loss of control over the lateral ligaments, there may be unusual varus. Sometimes small pieces of bone will break together with ligaments in the outer ankle, which is called avulsion fracture.

Injury of the medial ligament: There are not many cases caused by forceful outward turning (eversion) of the foot. Its concrete manifestation is similar to that of injury to the lateral ligaments, but in an opposite position and direction. It is marked by the pain in the medial ligaments, swelling and pain under pressure. When the foot turns outward, there will be pain in the medial ligaments and possibly avulsion fracture.

Target Acupoints

Legs: Kunlun (BL 60) and Taixi (KI 3) in coordination, Shangqiu (SP 5), Jiexi (ST 41), Sanyinjiao (SP 6) and Juegu in coordination, Qiuxu (GB 40).

Recommended Massage

1. Kunlun Point and Taixi Point in Coordination
Location: Kunlun point is in a cavity directly in the rear of the lateral malleolus. Taixi point is in a cavity between the medial malleolus and Achilles tendon.

Method: Sit upright. Use the thumb to press the Kunlun point forcefully on the same side, with the index finger pressing the Taixi point 20 to 30 times, until you cannot bear it. Pregnant women should not undertake this massage.

Effect: Chiefly serve to cure headache, visual dizziness, stiff neck, lumbar tingling, tinnitus, sore throat, insomnia, frequent urination, bed-wetting, menstrual disorder, ankle swelling with pain, ankle sprain, asthma, nephritis and cystitis.

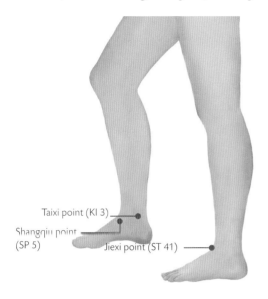

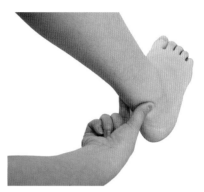

Kunlun point and Taixi point in coordination.

Location of the Taixi, Shangqiu and Jiexi points.

2. Pressing and Kneading the Jiexi Point

Location: In the middle at the front of the ankle.

Method: Sit upright and place the calf on the thigh of the opposite side. Use the thumb to forcefully press and knead the point 20 to 30 times, until tingling and distension are felt as the best effect.

Effect: Prevent and cure ankle sprain, foot arch droop, leg numbness, head-face edema, headache, dizziness, panic, abdominal distension and constipation.

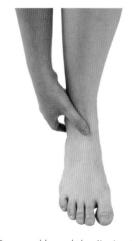

Press and knead the Jiexi point.

3. Pressing and Kneading the Shangqiu Point

Location: In a cavity midway between the tuberositas ossis navicularis and the inner ankle tip.

Method: Sit upright. Use the thumb to press and knead the Shangqiu point, with the rest of the fingers grasping the back of the foot. Move for about two minutes, until tingling and distension are felt as the best effect.

Effect: Cure abdominal pain and distension, diarrhea and ankle sprain.

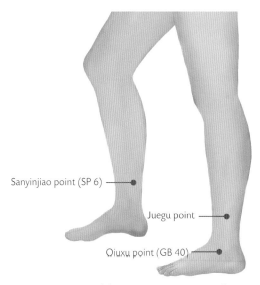

Sanyinjiao point (SP 6)

Juegu point

Qiuxu point (GB 40)

Location of the Sanyinjiao, Juegu and Qiuxu points.

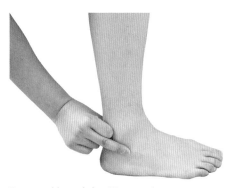

Press and knead the Qiuxu point.

4. Pressing and Kneading the Qiuxu Point

Location: In a cavity on the outer side of the extensor tendon.

Method: While squatting use the middle finger to press and knead the Qiuxu point of the affected side, with the thumb grasping the rear of the inner ankle, until you cannot bear the force.

Effect: Prevent and cure chest pain, cholecystitis, sciatica and leg paralysis as well as problems with the ankle joints and surrounding soft tissues.

5. Sanyinjiao Point and Juegu Point in Coordination

Location: The Sanyinjiao point is at the rear edge of the shinbone, three cun above the ankle. The Juegu point is three cun above the outer ankle tip.

Method: Sit upright, with the calf placed on the thigh of the other leg. Use the middle finger to forcefully press and knead the Juegu point of the affected side. At the same time use the thumb to press the Sanyinjiao point 20 to 30 times, until tingling and distension are felt as the best effect.

Effect: Treat sciatica, cerebrovascular diseases, hyperlipemia, high blood pressure, cervical spondylosis and chorea minor.

Tips

The thumb pad should be used immediately to stop bleeding after ankle sprain. When the pain is not so severe and there is no convulsion in the muscles on either side of the ankle, three tests should be undertaken (varus or valgus stress tests and drawer test) in order to ascertain if ligaments are completely torn.

If ligaments are torn or there is bone fracture, the patient should be sent to the hospital directly after the injured part has been stabilized and bandaged.

30 | Achilles Tendinitis

Common among people who undertake athletic activities, it is mostly due to inadequate preparation before hand, resulting in the sprain of the Achilles tendon at the moment of a sudden jump or sprint. Otherwise the injury may occur gradually, caused by extensive repeated training.

Symptoms

Achilles tendinitis is featured by pain in the Achilles tendon. It usually attacks at the beginning of athletic activities, but the pain diminishes during activity. Tension of the Achilles tendon is chiefly marked by pain in the heel in the early morning. There will be some swelling when it becomes serious.

Target Acupoints

Legs: Pain point, Sanyinjiao (SP 6) and Juegu in coordination, Kunlun (BL 60) and Taixi (KI 3) in coordination, Chengshan (BL 57).

Recommended Massage

1. Pressing and Kneading the Pain Point
Location: The pain point in the Achilles tendon.

    Method: Sit upright. Use the pad of the thumb and index finger to press and knead the point for three to five minutes.

    Effect: Eliminate adhesion and ease pain.

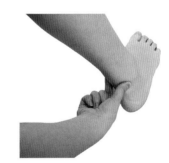

Press and knead the pain point.

2. Pressing the Chengshan Point
Location: In a cavity in the middle of the rear of the lower leg, at the top of the depression between the two muscles of the calf.

    Method: Sit upright. Use the thumb to press the Chengshan point for one minute, until some tingling and distension are felt as the best effect.

    Effect: Chiefly serve to cure calf muscle convulsion, sciatica, waist-back pain, leg paralysis, hemorrhoids, archoptosis and constipation.

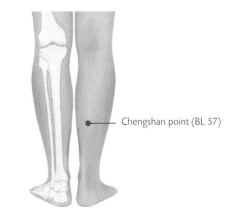

Chengshan point (BL 57)

Location of the Chengshan point.

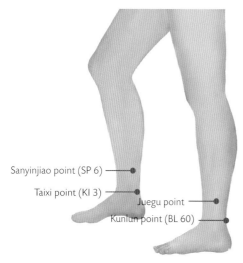

Sanyinjiao point (SP 6)

Taixi point (KI 3)

Juegu point

Kunlun point (BL 60)

Location of the Sanyinjiao, Taixi, Juegu and Kunlun points.

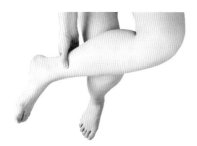

Sanyinjiao point and Juegu point in coordination.

3. Sanyinjiao Point and Juegu Point in Coordination

Location: The Sanyinjiao point is at the rear edge of the shinbone, three cun above the ankle. The Juegu point is three cun above the outer ankle tip.

Method: Sit upright, with the calf placed on the thigh of the other leg. Use the middle finger to forcefully press and knead the Juegu point of the affected side. At the same time use the thumb to press the Sanyinjiao point 20 to 30 times, until tingling and distension are felt as the best effect.

Effect: Treat sciatica, cerebrovascular diseases, hyperlipemia, high blood pressure, cervical spondylosis and chorea minor.

4. Kunlun Point and Taixi Point in Coordination

Location: Kunlun point is in a cavity directly in the rear of the lateral malleolus. Taixi point is in a cavity between the medial malleolus and Achilles tendon.

Method: Sit upright. Use the thumb to press the Kunlun point forcefully on the same side, with the index finger pressing the Taixi point 20 to 30 times, until you cannot bear it. Pregnant women should not undertake this massage.

Effect: Chiefly serve to cure headache, visual dizziness, stiff neck, lumbar tingling, tinnitus, sore throat, insomnia, frequent urination, bed-wetting, menstrual disorder, ankle swelling with pain, ankle sprain, asthma, nephritis and cystitis.

Tips
- Avoid aggressive activities and rest fully.
- Apply an ice compress to the injured part several times a day, for no more than 20 minutes each time.
- The swelling may lead to loss of movement in the injured joints. A binding or an elastic bandage can be used on the swollen part until the swelling disappears.

31 | Heel Pain

This pain occurring at the bottom of the heel is often seen among middle-aged people. It is mostly related to trauma and strain. Specifically it is caused by pathological changes in the bone, joints, bursa mucosa and fascia. Heel pain is often marked by a spur of the heel bone, fat pad inflammation under the heel, bone membrane inflammation of the heel bone, and tendon membrane inflammation.

Heel pain is divided into true heel pain and pseudo heel pain. Patients with true heel pain suffer from a heel spur. Patients with pseudo heel pain are free from heel spurs, but have continuous pain in the heel as well as heaviness and weakness in both legs.

Most patients have no history of obvious trauma, so this injury is often overlooked and timely treatment delayed.

Symptoms

It features severe pain in the heel. The painful part is restricted with an obvious pain point. Typically patients feel more pain when standing up or walking after getting up from the bed in the morning. The pain will be alleviated after walking for a short while, but there will be pain again when patients walk after rest.

Target Acupoints

Legs: Pain point, Qiuxu (GB 40), Sanyinjiao (SP 6), Kunlun (BL 60) and Taixi (KI 3) in coordination, Xuanzhong (GB 39).

Recommended Massage

1. Pressing and Kneading the Pain Point

Location: Painful part of the heel.

Method: With a hollow fist, use the index finger to press and knead the most painful part of the heel for three to five minutes, proceeding from light to heavy force, until some tingling and distension are felt.

Effect: Ease pain.

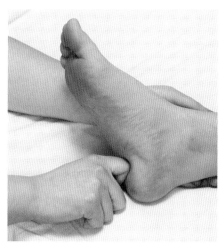

Press and knead the paint point.

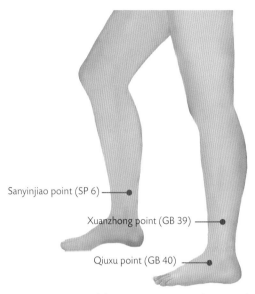

Sanyinjiao point (SP 6)

Xuanzhong point (GB 39)

Qiuxu point (GB 40)

Location of the Sanyinjiao, Xuanzhong and Qiuxu points.

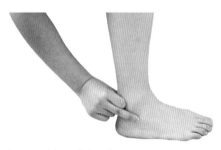

Press and knead the Qiuxu point.

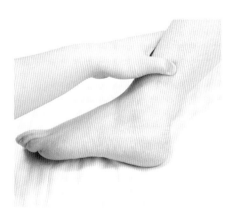

Press and knead the Xuanzhong point.

2. Pressing and Kneading the Qiuxu Point

Location: In a cavity on the outer side of the extensor tendon.

Method: While squatting use the middle finger to press and knead the Qiuxu point of the affected side outward for two minutes with the thumb attached to the rear of the inner ankle until you cannot bear the force exerted.

Effect: Prevent and cure chest pain, cholecystitis, sciatica, lower-limb paralysis and diseases of the surrounding soft tissues.

3. Pressing and Kneading the Sanyinjiao Point

Location: At the rear edge of the shinbone, three cun above the ankle.

Method: Sit upright and place one shin on the opposite thigh. Use the thumb to press, rub and knead the Sanyinjiao point for about two minutes until tingling and distension are felt in the part concerned as the best effect.

Effect: Cure insomnia, palpitation, high blood pressure, menstrual disorder, dysmenorrhea, impotence and nocturnal emission.

4. Pressing and Kneading the Xuanzhong Point

Location: In a cavity three cun above the outer ankle tip.

Method: Sit upright. Use the thumb to press the Xuanzhong point for about two minutes, until some tingling and distension are felt as the best effect.

Effect: Do away with liver and bone-marrow heat, relax tendons, soothe the liver and benefit the kidneys.

5. Kunlun Point and Taixi Point in Coordination

Location: Kunlun point is in a cavity directly in the rear of the lateral malleolus. Taixi point is in a cavity between the medial malleolus and Achilles tendon.

Method: Sit upright. Use the thumb and index finger to forcefully press the Kunlun point and Taixi point opposite respectively 20 to 30 times, until you cannot bear the force exerted. Prohibited for pregnant women.

Effect: Chiefly serve to cure headache, visual dizziness, stiff neck, lumbar tingling, tinnitus, sore throat, insomnia, frequent urination, bed-wetting, menstrual disorder, ankle swelling with pain, ankle sprain, asthma, nephritis and cystitis.

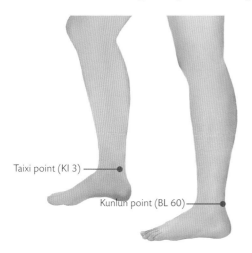

Taixi point (KI 3)

Kunlun point (BL 60)

Kunlun point and Taixi point in coordination.

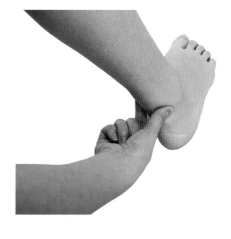

Press the Kunlun and Taixi points.

Tips

Pseudo heel pain can be prevented through these steps:
- Pay attention to keeping the heel warm.
- Avoid walking too much or standing too long.
- Take a foot bath in warm water or apply a hot compress to the feet before going to bed.
- Wear soft sole shoes.
- People with flat feet should avoid excessive movement and should wear corrective shoes.

32 | Rheumatoid Arthritis

It is a chronic systematic autoimmune disease, chiefly marked by synovitis, which is inflammation of the synovial membrane of the joints. It is most often seen among middle-aged women. Synovitis attacks continuously and repeatedly, resulting in damage to the cartilage, functional impediments of the joints and even physical disability.

Symptoms

Typical patients often experience gradual attack within several weeks or several months. This is marked by pain, swelling and stiffness in the fingers, palm and wrist joints, accompanied by general malaise, weakness, low fever, lack of appetite and reduction of weight.

Arthritis takes place repeatedly or develops continuously, affecting a number of joints with a distribution of left and right symmetry. The affected joints suffer from pain, swelling, pain of pressure and stiffness. Symptoms are most obvious after the patient gets up from the bed in the morning, but less serious after the patient moves around.

The movement of the affected joints is restricted due to continuous swelling. Those with light cases find it difficult to handle meticulous movements such as threading a needle and buttoning. Those with serious cases fail to complete daily movements such as washing the face and putting on clothes, leading to obvious decline in quality of life. Patients in the advanced stage have fixed joints due to malformation and rigidity. The most common case is that the palm is deformed, which may be called a "swan neck" as translated from the Chinese term.

Target Acupoints

Shoulder, back and waist: Zhishi (BL 52).
Chest and abdomen: Huangshu (KI 16).
Legs: Ququan (LV 8).

Recommended Massage

1. Pressing the Zhishi Point
Location: Three cun away from the spinous process of the second lumbar vertebra.
   Method: Lie down on the stomach. Use both thumbs to press it for two minutes.
   Effect: Treat nocturnal emission, impotence, difficult urination, edema, waist-back tingling and pain, lumbar muscle strain, sciatica, testicular swelling, pain, vaginal pain, indigestion, nausea and vomiting.

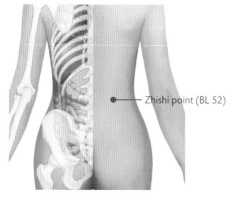

Zhishi point (BL 52)

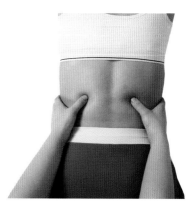

Press the Zhishi point.

2. Pressing the Huangshu Point

Location: At the point 0.5 cun away from the navel.

Method: Lie on the back with knees bent. Use overlapped middle fingers to press the point on one side for about three minutes.

Effect: Chiefly serve to cure pain around the navel, vomiting, abdominal distension, dysentery, diarrhea, constipation, hernia, menstrual disorder and lumbar-spine pain.

3. Pressing and Kneading Ququan Point

Location: With the knee bent, in the medial surface of the inner side of the knee.

Method: Sit upright. Use the index finger to press the Ququan point for two minutes, proceeding from light to heavy force.

Effect: Cure difficult urination, nocturnal emission, itches in the genital area and knee pain.

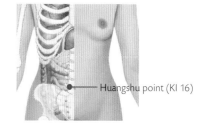

Huangshu point (KI 16)

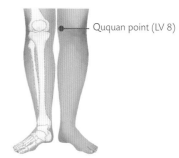

Ququan point (LV 8)

Location of the Huangshu and Ququan points.

Tips

- Try to reduce burden on the joints as well as violent movement to delay the process of pathological changes.
- Obese people should reduce weight to alleviate burden on the joints.
- In case of pathological changes in the legs, the patient can use a cane to reduce burden on the joints.
- In the period of morbidity, the patient should take anti-inflammation and analgesic medicine, after meals when possible.
- The affected joints should be protected by clothing or wraps, and the patient should pay attention to climatic changes, avoiding dampness or catching a cold.

33 | Hiccups

This is caused by incontrollable and convulsive contraction of the diaphragm. Alternatively it is the noise caused by semi-opening of the glottis within the throat. Hiccups will stop mostly within a few minutes.

Symptoms

Temporary hiccups will occur when one is irritated by the cold, eats or drinks too much or too fast, or consumes dry and hard food. The sleep, eating and work of people of with light cases will be affected, while the heart and lungs may be affected in people with serious cases. Correct massage, once mastered, can quickly control hiccups.

Target Acupoints

Head and neck: Cuanzhu (BL 2).
Chest and abdomen: Tiantu (RN 22), Danzhong (RN 17), Zhongwan (RN 12).
Arms: Neiguan (PC 6), Zhongkui (EX-UE 4), Hegu (LI 4).
Legs: Zusanli (ST 36).

Recommended Massage

1. Pressing the Cuanzhu Point
Location: In a cavity where the inner eyebrow starts.

Method: Use the pad of the middle finger to press the Cuanzhu point on the affected side. When there is a sense of tingling and distension, gradually increase force until tingling and distension radiate to the eyes, pressing for about two minutes in total.

Effect: It has a very good effect on eye tearing, dizziness, visual fatigue, eye edema, conjunctivitis, cheek pain, headache and high blood pressure. The Cuanzhu point is also often used in facial beauty treatment.

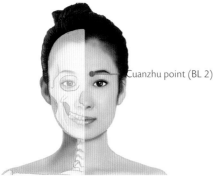
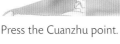
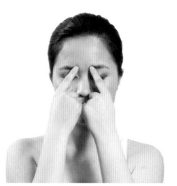

Cuanzhu point (BL 2)

Press the Cuanzhu point.

2. Pressing and Kneading the Zhongwan Point

Location: In between the lower part of the sternum and the navel.

Method: Sit upright or lie on the back. Use the middle or index finger to press the point for 30 seconds. Then continue to press and knead it for about two minutes, until distension and numbness are felt as the best effect.

Effect: As the most common acupoint used to cure diseases of the digestive system, it serves to cure stomachalgia, gastric convulsion, gastric ulcer, gastritis, hyperacidity, stomach atony, gastroptosis, nausea, vomiting, indigestion, abdominal pain, diarrhea and constipation.

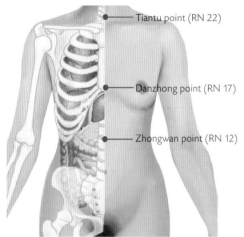
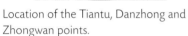

Location of the Tiantu, Danzhong and Zhongwan points.

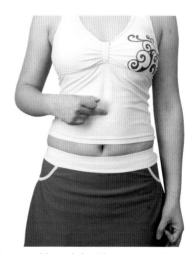

Press and knead the Zhongwan point.

3. Pressing the Tiantu Point

Location: Right in the middle of the cavity above the suprasternal fossa, just between the collarbones.

Method: Sit upright. Use the index fingertip of the left hand to press the Tiantu point, staying still for one minute after moving from the rear margin of the presternum downward. The force of massage is not supposed to affect the breathing of the patient.

Effect: Treat asthma, hiccups, cough, loss of speech, sore throat, thyromegaly, globus hystericus, cough with infection, bronchial asthma, bronchitis, pharyngitis and tonsillitis.

4. Palm Kneading the Danzhong Point

Location: Directly in the middle of the chest between the nipples.

Method: Sit upright or lie on the back. Use the thenar eminence of the left hand or palm heel to knead the Danzhong point for two minutes. Then use the thenar eminence of the right hand or palm heel to do it for two minutes, until distension and numbness are felt, radiating to the chest as the best effect.

Effect: Cure difficulty in breathing, cough, chest pain, hyperplasia of the mammary glands, breast pain, lactation problems, palpitation and obesity.

5. Pressing the Neiguan and Waiguan Points

Location: Between the two tendons about two cun above the wrist joint bend.

Method: Bend the forearm halfway. Use the thumb tip of one hand to press the Neiguan point while using the index or middle finger to press the Waiguan point, pressing inward 20 to 30 times.

Effect: Cure continuous hiccups, nausea, agitation, anxiety, palpitation, angina, chest distress, chest pain, coronary heart disease, insomnia, and gastric and intestinal neurosis.

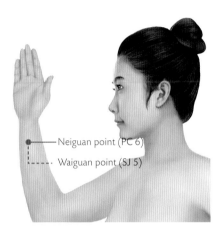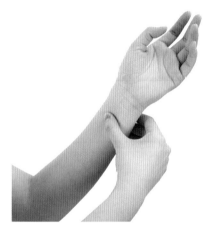

Press the Neiguan and Waiguan points.

6. Pinching and Kneading the Hegu Point

Location: In the highest point on the back of the hand between the thumb base and the base of the index finger (in the webbing between the two fingers).

Method: Use the thumb tip of one hand to pinch the Hegu point on the other hand for about one minute, and continue pinching and kneading for about two minutes, until some tingling and distension are felt as the best effect.

Effect: Treat facioplegia, trigeminal pain, facial paralysis, deviated mouth and eyes (facial paralysis), rhinitis, headache, toothache, acne, visual fatigue, sore throat, tinnitus and hiccups.

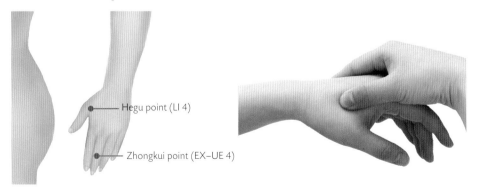

Location of the Hegu and Zhongkui points.   Pinch and knead the Hegu point.

7. Pressing and Kneading the Zhongkui Point

Location: In the middle near the interphalangeal joint on the rear side of the middle finger.

Method: Make a fist. Use the index finger to press and knead the point for about three minutes.

Effect: Cure dysphagia, vomiting, lack of appetite and hiccups.

8. Pressing and Kneading the Zusanli Point

Location: About three cun below the knee on the outer side of the tibia.

Method: Sit upright. Use two thumbs to press the Zusanli point of both sides outward, with the rest of the fingers grasping the rear of the calf, repeating 20 to 40 times, until tingling and distension are felt as the best effect.

Effect: Cure diarrhea, abdominal pain, lack of appetite, constipation, hiccups, vomiting, anemia, low blood pressure, menopause syndrome and waist-leg pain.

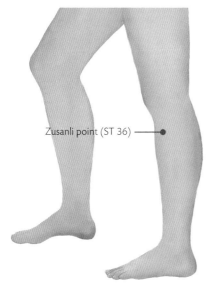
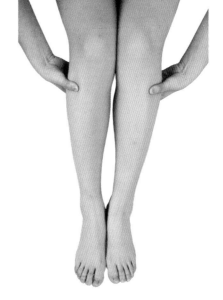

Zusanli point (ST 36)

Press and knead the Zusanli point.

Tips

Continuous hiccupping lasting for days is likely to be the symptom of gastric, diaphragm, heart or liver diseases, or tumor. Therefore timely diagnosis and medical treatment are required.

34 Nausea and Vomiting

Gastric diseases are mostly accompanied by nausea and vomiting. However nausea and vomiting are among the symptoms of a number of diseases, such as gastric ulcer, duodenal ulcer and gastritis.

Symptoms

At the beginning there is discomfort in the stomach, followed by nausea and vomiting. The most common occurrence is that the patient spits up undigested food. Some patients spit up yellowish-green bitter water.

Vomiting in pregnant women is normal, requiring no treatment in general. However timely treatment is still needed if it is serious.

Target Acupoints

Chest and abdomen: Tiantu (RN 22), Tianshu (ST 25), Zhongwan (RN 12).
Arms: Neiguan (PC 6).
Legs: Liangqiu (ST 34), Gongsun (SP 4), Zusanli (ST 36), Yanglingquan (GB 34).

Recommended Massage

1. Pressing the Tiantu Point
Location: Right in the middle of the cavity above the suprasternal fossa, just between the collarbones.

Method: Sit upright. Use the thumb tip of the left hand to press the Tiantu point, staying still for one minute after moving from the rear margin of the presternum downward. The force of massage is not supposed to affect the breathing of the patient.

Effect: Treat asthma, hiccups, cough, loss of speech, sore throat, thyromegaly, globus hystericus, cough with infection, bronchial asthma, bronchitis, pharyngitis and tonsillitis.

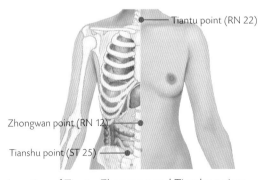

Location of Tiantu, Zhongwan and Tianshu points.

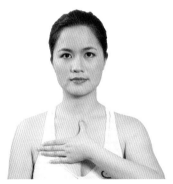

Press the Tiantu point.

2. Pressing and Kneading the Tianshu Point

Location: About two cun horizontally away from the navel.

Method: Sit upright or lie on the back. Use two thumbs to press the Tianshu points on both sides for two minutes, until some tingling and distension are felt, ideally radiating to the entire abdomen.

Effect: Cure abdominal distension and pain, nausea, vomiting, constipation, diarrhea, menstrual disorder and dysmenorrhea.

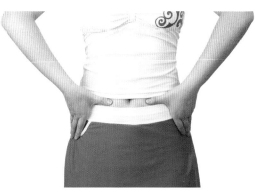

Press and knead the Tianshu point.

3. Pressing and Kneading the Zhongwan Point

Location: In between the lower part of the sternum and the navel.

Method: Lie on the back or sit upright. First use the index or middle finger to press the point for 30 seconds. Then continue to press and knead it for two minutes, until some tingling and distension are felt.

Effect: Cure abdominal pain and distension, diarrhea, acid regurgitation, vomiting and constipation.

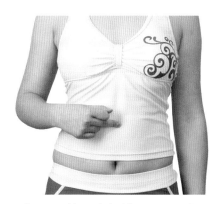

Press and knead the Zhongwan point.

4. Pressing the Neiguan and Waiguan Points

Location: Between the two tendons about two cun above the wrist joint bend.

Method: With the forearm bent halfway, use the thumb tip of one hand to press the Neiguan point in the other forearm, while using the index or middle finger to press the Waiguan point. Press them simultaneously 20 to 30 times, until tingling and distension are felt as the best effect.

Effect: Cure vomiting, hiccups, chest distress, chest pain, insomnia, agitation, palpitation, gastritis, gastric ulcer, heat-stroke and migraine.

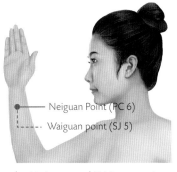

Neiguan Point (PC 6)

Waiguan point (SJ 5)

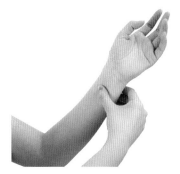

Press the Neiguan and Waiguan points.

5. Pressing and Kneading the Liangqiu Point

Location: With the knee bent, on the outer edge of the thigh, two cun above the outer upper margin of the patella.

Method: Sit upright with knees bent. Use two thumbs to press the point for about one minute. If the symptoms fail to disappear, you should press and knead for another two minutes.

Effect: Treat diseases of the digestive system such as gastric convulsion, gastritis, diarrhea and vomiting; diseases of gynecology and obstetrics such as mastitis and dysmenorrhea; and orthopedic issues such as rheumatic arthritis, suprapatellar bursitis, chondromalacia patellae and pathological changes in the knee joints.

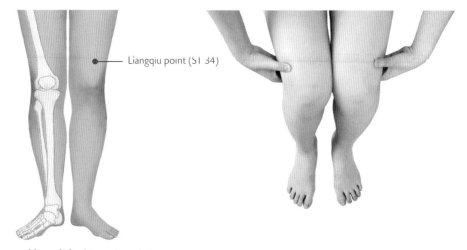

Press and knead the Liangqiu point.

6. Pressing and Kneading the Gongsun Point

Location: At the point of the frontal lower part at the base of the first metatarsal bone.

Method: Sit upright. Use the thumb tip to press and knead the point for two minutes and then continue to press it for another 30 seconds, until tingling and distension are felt as the best effect.

Effect: Treat acute gastritis, gastric convulsion, intestinal convulsion, acute enteritis, nervous vomiting, diaphragm spasm, the aftereffect of myocarditis, pleurisy, peritonitis, head-face edema, epilepsy, ascites due to cirrhosis, malaria, leg paralysis and inflammation at the inguinal lymph nodes.

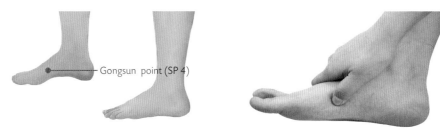

Press and knead the Gongsun point.

7. Pressing and Kneading the Zusanli Point
Location: About three cun below the knee on the outer side of the tibia.

Method: Sit upright. Use both thumbs to press the point on both sides, with the four fingers alongside the outer side of the lower leg, pressing and kneading outward 20 to 40 times, until some tingling and distension are felt as the best effect.

Effect: Cure nausea, vomiting, diarrhea, gastric and abdominal pain, lack of appetite and constipation.

8. Pressing and Kneading the Yanglingquan Point
Location: On the outer side of the shin in a notch at the front lower part of the fibula.

Method: Sit upright. Use the thumb tip to press the Yanglingquan point of the affected side, while putting the other four fingers at the rear of the lower leg, pressing and kneading for two to three minutes with slightly heavy force until some tingling and distension are obviously felt. Some patients will feel radiative numbness toward the outer side of the calf.

Effect: Treat jaundice, rib pain, bitter taste in the mouth, vomiting and acid regurgitation from liver and gallbladder problems related to gastric diseases, knee swelling and pain, lower limb paralysis and numbness, knee joint problems and febrile convulsion.

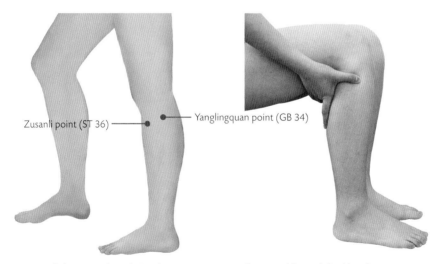

Location of the Zusanli and Yanglingquan points.   Press and knead the Yanglingquan point.

Tips

Before the cause of the disease is determined, no antiemetic medicine should be taken so as to prevent improper treatment. In other words the cause of the disease should be determined first before targeted treatment is applied.

35 | Lack of Appetite

Appetite is a normal physiological need for eating food. The decline or disappearance of such a need is called the lack of appetite.

There are many causes, such as fatigue and tension, which will result in temporary lack of appetite. In addition drinking or eating too much, reducing weight or some diseases may lead to lack of appetite.

Symptoms

The lack of appetite usually occurs when one is not in a good mood, lacks enough sleep, feels tired and doesn't eat varied foods. These phenomena generally last for a short time. With the above-mentioned reasons eliminated, people will restore appetite quickly.

However if the lack of appetite occurs without any reason and/or lasts quite a long time, one should be alert since it is can be an early signal of some kinds of diseases.

Target Acupoints

Shoulder, back and waist: Weishu (BL 21), Pishu (BL 20).
Chest and abdomen: Liangmen (ST 21), Zhongwan (RN 12), Tianshu (ST 25), Xiawan (RN 10).
Legs: Zusanli (ST 36), Yongquan (KI 1).

Recommended Massage

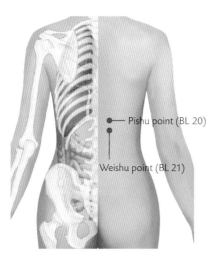

Pishu point (BL 20)

Weishu point (BL 21)

Location of the Pishu and Weishu points.

1. Pressing and Kneading the Weishu Point
Location: About 1.5 cun below the spinous process of the twelfth thoracic vertebra.

Method: Sit or stand. Use the middle fingers to press and knead the Weishu point of both sides (with the thumb against the ribs) forcefully for two minutes. Alternately make a fist and use the protruding index knuckle to press and knead it for two minutes. Or with a loose fist, press and rub the point for two minutes. In all cases some tingling and distension are felt as the best effect.

Effect: Treat all kinds of diseases and symptoms of the digestive system, such as acute gastritis, chronic gastritis, gastroptosis, stomach atony, abdominal distension, abdominal pain, lack of appetite, nausea and vomiting.

2. Pressing and Kneading the Pishu Point

Location: At the point 1.5 cun away horizontally from the eleventh thoracic vertebra.

Method: Sit or stand. Use both middle fingers to press the Pishu point, with the thumb against the ribs, forcefully pressing and kneading for two minutes. Or with a clenched fist, use the index knuckle to press and knead the Pishu point for two minutes. Alternatively you may use a hollow fist to knead and rub it for two minutes, until some tingling and distension are felt.

Effect: Cure nausea, vomiting, abdominal distension, diarrhea, hemafecia (bloody stool) and jaundice.

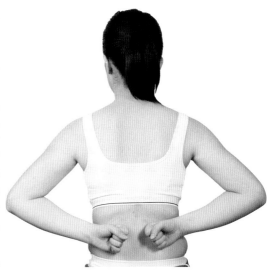

Press and knead the Pishu point.

3. Pressing and Kneading the Liangmen Point

Location: Four cun above the navel and two cun away from it.

Method: Lie on the back. Use the index finger to press and knead the point for about two minutes, proceeding from light to heavy force.

Effect: Benefit the spleen and stomach, help digestion, stimulate appetite, and cure gastric pain, vomiting and hyperactive bowel sounds.

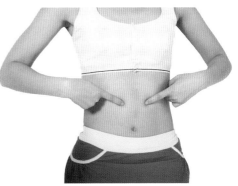

Press and knead the Liangmen point.

4. Pressing and Kneading the Zhongwan Point

Location: In between the lower part of the sternum and the navel.

Method: Lie on the back or sit upright. First use the index or middle finger to press the point for 30 seconds. Then continue to press and knead it for two minutes, until some tingling and distension are felt.

Effect: Cure abdominal pain and distension, diarrhea, acid regurgitation, vomiting and constipation.

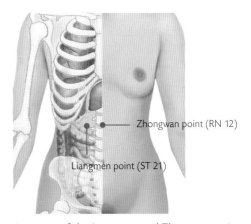

Zhongwan point (RN 12)

Liangmen point (ST 21)

Location of the Liangmen and Zhongwan points.

5. Pressing and Kneading the Tianshu Point

Location: About two cun horizontally away from the navel.

Method: Sit upright or lie on the back. Use two thumbs to press the point on both sides for 30 seconds. Then continue to press and knead for another two minutes, until some tingling and distension are felt, ideally radiating to the entire abdomen.

Effect: Cure abdominal distension and pain, nausea, vomiting, constipation, diarrhea, menstrual disorder and dysmenorrhea.

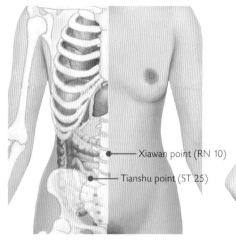

Xiawan point (RN 10)

Tianshu point (ST 25)

Location of the Xiawan and Tianshu points.

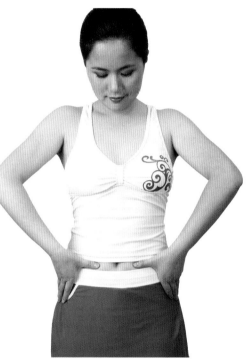

Press and knead the Tianshu point.

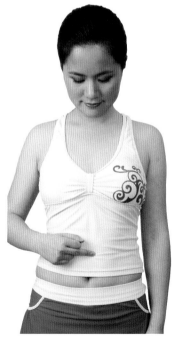

Press and knead the Xiawan point.

6. Pressing and Kneading the Xiawan Point

Location: 2 cun above the navel.

Method: Lie on the back or sit upright. First use the index or middle finger to press the point for 30 seconds. Then continue to press and knead it for another two minutes, until some tingling and distension are felt.

Effect: Cure abdominal distension and pain, diarrhea, acid reflux, vomiting and constipation.

7. Pressing and Kneading the Zusanli Point

Location: About three cun below the knee on the outer side of the tibia.

Method: Sit upright. Use both thumbs to press the point on both sides, with the four fingers alongside the outer side of the lower leg, pressing and kneading outward 20 to 40 times, until some tingling and distension are felt as the best effect.

Effect: Cure nausea, vomiting, diarrhea, stomachalgia, abdominal pain, lack of appetite and constipation.

8. Pressing and Kneading the Yongquan Point

Location: In a depression in the front of the sole of the foot, about one-third of the way down from the toes.

Method: Sit while stretching one leg straight, with the other leg placed on the knee of the stretched leg. Use one hand to hold the foot back while using the thumb of the other hand to press and knead the point in a small area vertically for two minutes.

Effect: Treat pain and distension of the sole of the foot, pale or peeling foot skin, fever, nasal discomfort and allergy, diarrhea, agitation, dizziness, insomnia, constipation and difficult urination. Some massage serves to speed up blood circulation in the foot and promote metabolism.

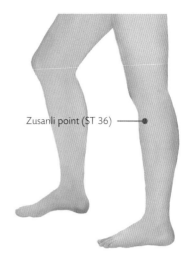

Zusanli point (ST 36)

Location of the Zusanli point.

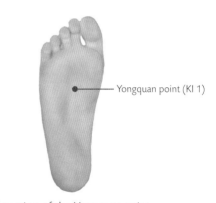

Yongquan point (KI 1)

Location of the Yongquan point.

Tips

There are several diseases that are likely to cause lack of appetite:

It is usually anemia if the lack of appetite is accompanied by dizziness, seeing stars, fatigue, abdominal distension, palpitation, and pale lips and fingernails.

It is usually acute or chronic gastritis or ulcer if accompanied by nausea, vomiting, and fullness, distension and pain of the upper abdomen as well as frequent acid reflux and belching.

It is usually liver cirrhosis if accompanied by the loss of weight, weakness, nausea, abdominal distension, diarrhea and a gray tinge to the face.

One should see a doctor as soon as possible if he/she has these symptoms.

36 | Stomachalgia

This pain attacks chiefly near the stomach close to the heart.

A common disease, it can be caused by many other diseases, such as acute and chronic gastritis, gastric ulcer, duodenal ulcer and neurosis, as well as prolapse of gastric mucosa, gastroptosis, pancreatitis, cholecystitis and gallstones.

Gastritis is mostly associated with diet, such as drinking and eating too much, or being either very full or very hungry.

Symptoms

It attacks often due to the cold weather, catching a cold and eating cold food. The pain is sometimes accompanied by a cold feeling in the stomach, but eases after having been warmed up.

Target Acupoints

Shoulder, back and waist: Weishu (BL 21).
Chest and abdomen: Shangwan (RN 13), Liangmen (ST 21), Zhongwan (RN 12).
Arms: Neiguan (PC 6).
Legs: Liangqiu (ST 34), Zusanli (ST 36), Gongsun (SP 4).

Recommended Massage

1. Pressing and Kneading the Weishu Point
Location: About 1.5 cun below the spinous process of the twelfth thoracic vertebra.

Method: Sit or stand. Use the middle fingers to press and knead the Weishu point of both sides (with the thumb against the ribs) forcefully for two minutes.

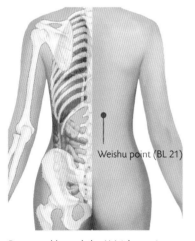
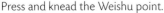

Weishu point (BL 21)

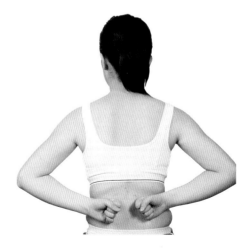

Press and knead the Weishu point.

Alternately make a fist and use the protruding index knuckle to press and knead it for two minutes. Or with a loose fist, press and rub the point for two minutes. In all cases some tingling and distension are felt as the best effect.

Effect: Treat all kinds of diseases and symptoms of the digestive system, such as acute gastritis, chronic gastritis, gastroptosis, stomach atony, abdominal distension, abdominal pain, lack of appetite, nausea and vomiting.

2 . Pressing and Kneading the Liangmen Point

Location: Four cun above the navel and two cun away from it.

Method: Sit upright or lie on the back. Use the pad of the index finger to press and knead the point for three minutes, proceeding from light to heavy force.

Effect: Benefit spleen, stomach and digestion, as well as stimulate appetite while curing gastric pain, vomiting and hyperactive bowel sounds.

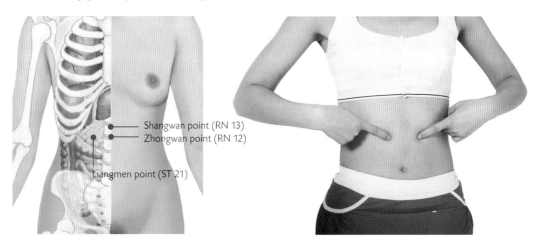

Location of the Liangmen, Shangwan and Zhongwan points.

Press and knead the Liangmen point.

3. Pressing and Kneading the Shangwan Point

Location: Five cun above the navel.

Method: Sit upright or lie on the back. Use the index or middle finger to press the point for one minute, and then continue to press and knead it for another two minutes.

Effect: Treat nausea, vomiting, indigestion, gastric pain, anorexia, abdominal distension and pain, cough with mucus, jaundice, hematemesis due to physical weakness, gastritis, gastric dilatation, phrenospasm and enteritis.

4. Pressing and Kneading the Zhongwan Point

Location: In between the lower part of the sternum and the navel.

Method: Lie on the back or sit upright. First use the index or middle finger to press the point for 30 seconds. Then continue to press and knead it for two minutes, until some tingling and distension are felt.

Effect: Cure abdominal pain and distension, diarrhea, acid regurgitation, vomiting and constipation.

5. Pressing the Neiguan and Waiguan points

Location: Between the two tendons about two cun above the wrist joint bend.

Method: With the forearm bent halfway, use the thumb tip of one hand to press the Neiguan point in the other forearm, while using the index or middle finger to press the Waiguan point. Press them simultaneously 20 to 30 times, until tingling and distension are felt as the best effect.

Effect: Treat continuous hiccups, nausea, agitation, anxiety, palpitation, angina pectoris, chest distress, chest pain, coronary heart disease, insomnia, gastric and intestinal neurosis.

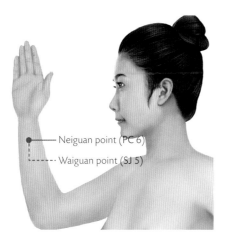
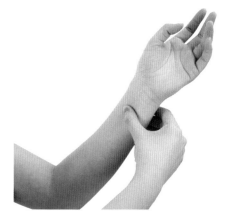

Press the Neiguan and Waiguan points.

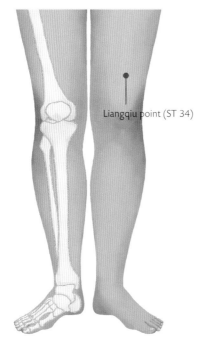

Location of the Liangqiu point.

6. Pressing and Kneading the Liangqiu Point

Location: With the knee bent, on the outer edge of the thigh, two cun above the outer upper margin of the patella.

Method: Sit with knees bent. Use the tips of both thumbs to press and knead the Liangqiu points on both sides for about one minute, which can stop stomachalgia at once. If the pain still attacks, press and knead it for another two minutes.

Effect: Treat diseases of the digestive system such as gastric convulsion, gastritis, diarrhea and vomiting; diseases of gynecology and obstetrics such as mastitis and dysmenorrhea; and orthopedic issues such as rheumatic arthritis, suprapatellar bursitis, chondromalacia patellae and pathological changes in the knee joints.

7. Pressing and Kneading the Zusanli Point

Location: About three cun below the knee on the outer side of the tibia.

Method: Sit upright. Use both thumbs to press the point on both sides, with the four fingers alongside the outer side of the lower leg, pressing and kneading outward 20 to 40 times, until some tingling and distension are felt as the best effect.

Effect: Treat diarrhea, abdominal pain and distension, lack of appetite, constipation, hiccups, vomiting, anemia, low blood pressure, menopause syndrome and waist-leg pain.

8. Pressing and Kneading the Gongsun Point

Location: At the point of the frontal lower part at the base of the first metatarsal bone.

Method: Sit upright. Use the thumb tip to press and knead the point for two minutes and then continue to press it for another 30 seconds, until tingling and distension are felt as the best effect.

Effect: Treat acute gastritis, gastric convulsion, intestinal convulsion, acute enteritis, nervous vomiting, diaphragm spasm, the aftereffect of myocarditis, pleurisy, peritonitis, head-face edema, epilepsy, ascites due to cirrhosis, malaria, leg paralysis and inflammation at the inguinal lymph nodes.

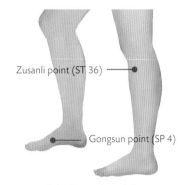

Location of the Zusanli and Gongsun points.

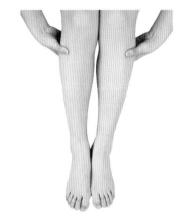

Press and knead the Zusanli point.

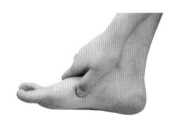

Press and knead the Gongsun point.

Tips

Other ways to alleviate the pain:
- Loosen the belt when the pain attacks, to make the abdomen comfortable.
- Try to wear comfortable and loose clothes to prevent the abdomen from being pressed.
- For those often suffering from acid reflux, it is better to sleep on the left side while raising the pillow.

37 | Constipation

It refers excrement congestion, which is caused by many reasons, such as sitting for a long time, lack of exercise, and inadequate intake of coarse fiber in the diet. On the whole women suffer from it more than men.

Symptoms

It is marked by lower defecating frequency, the extension of excrement discharge over more days, or dry excrement. It may involve difficult discharge despite the normal frequency of defection, or difficult discharge despite the normal state of the excrement.

Constipation sometimes goes together with abdominal pain, decline of appetite and nausea.

However some people defecate once every several days without any discomfort. In principle it cannot be regarded as constipation if there is no pain while defecating.

Target Acupoints

Shoulder, back and waist: Baliao (BL 31–34), Dachangshu (BL 25).
Chest and abdomen: Tianshu (ST 25), Daju (ST 27), Zhongwan (RN 12), Daheng (SP 15).
Arms: Zhigou (SJ 6).
Legs: Shangjuxu (ST 37), Taibai (SP 3).

Recommended Massage

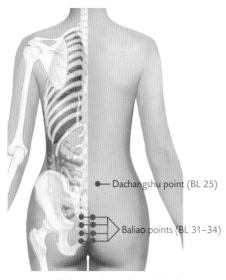

Location of the Dachangshu and Baliao points.

Dachangshu point (BL 25)
Baliao points (BL 31–34)

1. Kneading and Rubbing the Baliao Points

Location: There are eight Baliao points in total, four on each side of the sacral spine. These are the upper, secondary, middle and lower Baliao points. They are located respectively in the first, second, third and fourth posterior sacral foramina (opening between vertebrae).

Method: Sit upright. Use the palm to knead, or rub up and down, along the sacral vertebrae for about two minutes, until some tingling and distension are felt as the best effect.

Effect: Cure pain in the lumbosacral spine, constipation, distension and pain in the lower abdomen, pelvic inflammation, difficult urination, menstrual disorder and hemorrhoids.

2. Pressing and Kneading the Dachangshu Point

Location: About 1.5 cun away from the fourth lumbar vertebra on two sides.

Method: Sit or stand with arms akimbo. Use the thumb pad to press and knead the Dachangshu points on both sides for about two minutes. You can also make a fist to press with the index knuckle for one minute, until some tingling and distension are felt as the best effect.

Effect: Cure constipation, abdominal pain and distension, borborygmus, waist-back pain and premature ejaculation.

3. Pressing and Kneading the Tianshu Point

Location: About two cun horizontally away from the navel.

Method: Sit upright or lie on the back. Use two thumbs to press and knead the Tianshu points of both sides for two minutes, with the four fingers grasping the lateral waist, until some tingling and distension are felt, ideally radiating to the entire abdomen.

Effect: Cure abdominal distension and pain, nausea, constipation, diarrhea, menstrual disorder and dysmenorrhea.

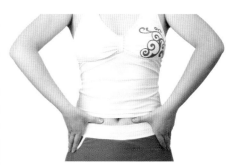

Press and knead the Tianshu point.

4. Pressing and Kneading the Daju Point

Location: Two cun below the navel, two cun away from the median line.

Method: Lie on the back with knees bent. Using the four fingers of both hands, press and knead it respectively.

Effect: Chiefly serve to cure distension of the lower abdomen, difficult urination, hernia, nocturnal emission, premature ejaculation, convulsion of the rectus abdominis, intestinal obstruction, cystitis and urinary retention.

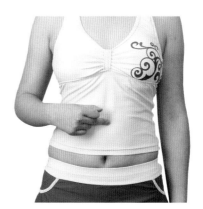

Press the Zhongwan point.

5. Pressing the Zhongwan Point

Location: In between the lower part of the sternum and the navel.

Method: Sit upright or lie on the back. First use the index or middle finger to press the point for 30 seconds. Then press and knead it for another two minutes, until some tingling and distension are felt as the best effect.

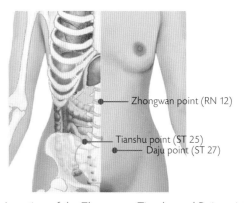

Zhongwan point (RN 12)

Tianshu point (ST 25)
Daju point (ST 27)

Location of the Zhongwan, Tianshu and Daju points.

Effect: Cure diseases of the digestive system such as constipation, abdominal distension and pain, diarrhea, borborygmus, vomiting and acid regurgitation, in addition to having a very good effect on curing visual dizziness, acne, decline of energy and neurasthenia.

6. Pressing and Kneading the Daheng Point
Location: Four cun away from the navel, in line with the nipple.

Method: Sit upright or lie on back. Use two thumbs to press and knead the Daheng point of the same side for 30 seconds, with the rest of the fingers grasping the lateral waist. Then continue for another two minutes, until some tingling and distension are felt, ideally radiating to the entire abdomen.

Effect: Cure spleen and stomach diseases such as abdominal pain, diarrhea and constipation.

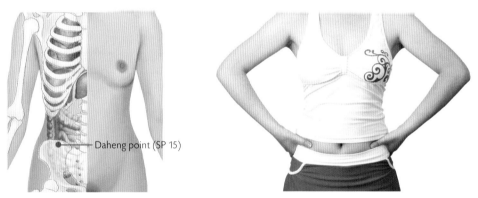

Daheng point (SP 15)

Press and knead the Daheng point.

7. Pressing and Kneading the Zhigou Point
Location: In a cavity about three cun above the back of the wrist, between the two bones of the forearm.

Method: Use the thumb to press and knead the Zhigou point for two minutes, until some tingling and distension are felt as the best effect.

Effect: Cure habitual constipation, rib pain, shoulder-arm tingling and pain, difficulty in passing urine and agalactia.

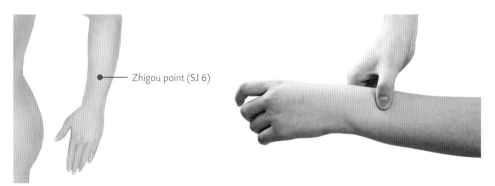

Zhigou point (SJ 6)

Press and knead the Zhigou point.

8. Pressing and Kneading the Shangjuxu Point

Location: One middle finger cun on the outside of the tibial crest. Three cun below the Zusanli point.

Method: Sit upright. Use two thumbs to press and knead the Shangjuxu point for two minutes, until some tingling and distension are felt as the best effect.

Effect: Treat diseases of the digestive system such as appendicitis, gastric and intestinal inflammation, diarrhea, dysentery, hernia, constipation and indigestion, in addition to curing aftereffects of cerebrovascular diseases, leg paralysis or spasm, and knee-joint swelling and pain.

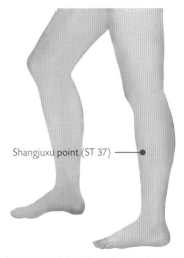

Shangjuxu point (ST 37)

Location of the Shangjuxu point.

9. Pushing the Taibai Point

Location: On the inside of the foot, near the ball of the foot at the first metatarsophalangeal joint.

Method: Sit upright, with one leg stretching straight and the other leg placed on the knee of the straightened leg. Use one hand to fix the ankle while using the thumb of the other hand to push from the foot tip to the ankle 30 to 40 times, centering around the Taibai point.

Effect: Chiefly serve to cure stomachalgia, abdominal distension, vomiting, hiccups, borborygmus, diarrhea, dysentery, constipation, dermatophytosis and anal fistula.

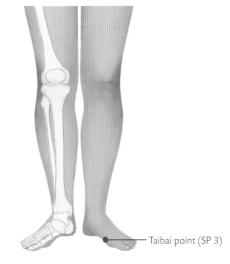

Taibai point (SP 3)

Location of the Taibai point.

Tips
- Drink a cup of boiled water or a cup of water with honey after getting up in the morning.
- Avoid eating hot and spicy food to prevent irritation.
- Eat more food with coarse fiber, such as lotus roots, celery and whole wheat.
- Take in a proper amount of fat to help movement of the intestinal tract.

38 | Colds

The cold is a kind of upper respiratory disease caused by virus, mixed infection or abnormal reaction. It takes place all year round, particularly in spring and winter or when resistance against diseases weakens. It is divided into the common cold and influenza (abbreviated as flu).

Common cold is a widespread respiratory disease mostly caused by a variety of viruses. Thirty to fifty percent are caused by a certain nasal virus. Though appearing mostly in winter, it occurs in any season. Viruses leading to the cold in different seasons are not the same.

Flu is a kind of acute infectious disease of the respiratory system caused by a flu virus that is found in the respiratory system of the patient. Such a virus can infect other people when the patient spreads saliva through coughing or sneezing.

Symptoms

The common cold mostly takes place in autumn and winter in two stages. The first stage sees sneezing, nasal congestion, runny nose, soreness and physical weakness. If not treated in a timely manner, it will develop into the second stage, which is marked by fever, headache, joint pain and cough.

Flu is also caused by a virus, the most common being influenza A. Flu occurs very violently at the beginning, marked by cold shivering, high fever, muscle soreness all over the body and headache. However other symptoms related to the upper respiratory system are milder.

Target Acupoints

Head and neck: Yingxiang (LI 20), Taiyang (EX-HN 5), Fengchi (GB 20), Fengfu (DU 16).
Shoulder, back and waist: Dazhui (DU 14), Feishu (BL 13), Fengmen (BL 12).
Chest and abdomen: Zhongfu (LU 1), Juque (RN 14).
Arms: Hegu (LI 4).

Recommended Massage

1. Pressing and Kneading the Yingxiang Point
Location: Beside the wing of the nose, 0.5 cun away, in the nasolabial groove.

Method: Sit upright or lie on the back. Place the pads of the index or middle fingers on the Yingxiang points on both sides to press, rub and knead for two minutes until tingling and distension are felt in the part concerned as the best effect.

Effect: Reinforce sense of smell while curing and preventing rhinitis and nasosinusitis, facioplegia and facial convulsion.

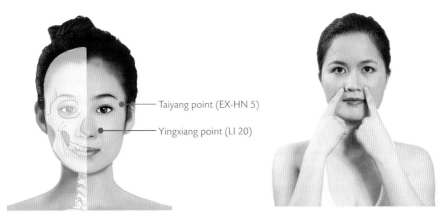

Location of the Taiyang and Yingxiang points.

Press and knead the Yingxiang point.

2. Pressing and Kneading the Taiyang Point

Location: In the depression about one cun behind the space between the outer tip of the brow and outer eye corner.

Method: Sit upright or lie on the back. Place both finger pads on the Taiyang points to press, rub and knead for two minutes until tingling and distension are felt in the part concerned as the best effect. If a larger area or more force is needed, the thenar eminences of both hands can do the job.

Effect: Treat cold, fever, headache, dizziness, red and swollen eyes with pain.

3. Pressing and Kneading the Fengchi Point

Location: In the depression on both sides of the large tendon behind the nape of the neck, next to the lower edge of the skull.

Method: Sit upright. Place both pads of the index and middle fingers on the Fengchi point to press, rub and knead for two minutes until tingling and distension are felt in the part concerned as the best effect.

Effect: Treat cold, fever, stiff and painful neck, headache, dizziness, red and swollen eyes with pain.

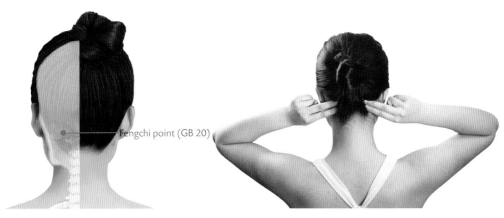

Press and knead the Fengchi point.

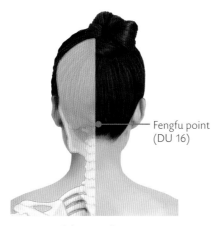

Location of the Fengfu point.

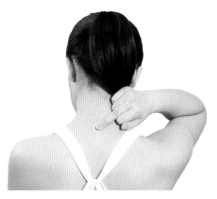

Press the Dazhui point.

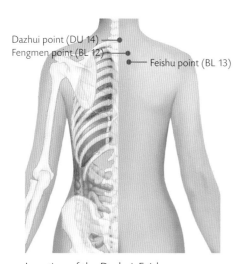

Location of the Dazhui, Feishu and Fengmen points.

4. Pressing and Kneading the Fengfu Point

Location: At the back of the head on the midline, one cun above the hairline in a notch.

Method: Sit upright. Use the thumb to press, rub and knead the Fengfu point for three minutes, proceeding from light to heavy force until tingling and distension are felt in the part concerned.

Effect: Channel meridians and collaterals, and eliminate cold, as well as ease headache, pressure in the head, fatigue all over the body, sneezing, runny nose, nasal congestion, fever and cold feeling caused by the cold.

5. Pressing the Dazhui Point

Location: Under the spinous process of the seventh cervical vertebrae.

Method: Sit upright. Use the tip of the middle finger to press the Dazhui point 20 or 30 times.

Effect: An important acupoint for health care, it serves to enhance the ability of preventing diseases, and to treat headache and neck pain, neck-shoulder syndrome, cervical spondylosis, fever, cold, asthma, malaria, chronic bronchitis, tuberculosis (TB) and epilepsy as well as cold limbs, shoulder-back cold pain and physical weakness caused by the lack of vital energy.

6. Pressing and Kneading the Feishu Point

Location: At the point 1.5 cun beside the third thoracic vertebra on the inner side of the scapula.

Method: Sit upright. First place the left palm heel on the Jianjing point on the right side, with the middle fingertip pressing, rubbing and kneading the Feishu point on the right side for two minutes. Then place the right palm heel on the Jianjing point on the left side, kneading until the part concerned feels hot as the best effect.

Effect: Treat cold, cough, bronchitis, asthma, spontaneous perspiration, night sweating and back tingling and pain.

7. Pressing and Kneading the Fengmen Point

Location: 1.5 cun below the spinous process of the second thoracic vertebra.

Method: Sit upright. Use the middle finger of the left hand to press, rub and knead the Fengmen point on the right side while using the middle finger of the right hand to press, rub and knead the Fengmen point on the left. Massage each Fengmen point for two minutes until you feel obvious tingling and distension in the part concerned as the best effect.

Effect: Chiefly serve to cure neck-back pain, cold and diseases of the respiratory system.

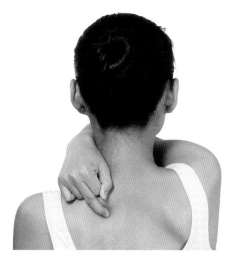

Press and knead the Fengmen point.

8. Pinching and Kneading the Hegu Point

Location: In the highest point on the back of the hand between the thumb base and the base of the index finger (in the webbing between these two fingers).

Method: Sit upright or lie on the back. Use the thumb to pinch and knead the Hegu point 10 to 20 times proceeding from light to heavy force, until you feel tingling and distension in the part concerned as the best effect. Pinching and kneading are applied to this acupoint on both hands alternately.

Effect: Cure cold, runny nose, toothache, acne, visual fatigue, sore throat, tinnitus and hiccups.

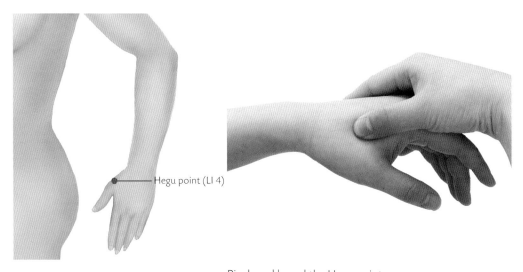

Hegu point (LI 4)

Pinch and knead the Hegu point.

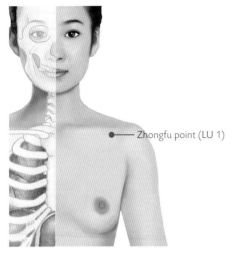

Location of the Zhongfu point.

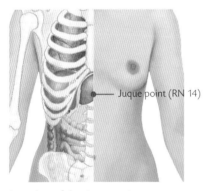

Location of the Juque point.

9. Pressing and Kneading the Zhongfu Point

Location: At the center of a notch below the S-shaped collarbone in front of the shoulder.

Method: Sit upright or lie on the back. Place the thumb tips on this acupoint on both sides, with the rest of the fingers on the chest. Press forcefully for about 30 seconds continuously, then knead for two minutes.

Effect: Cough will be alleviated with smooth breathing achieved at once. It also serves to treat tracheitis, bronchial asthma, pneumonia, chest pain and shoulder-back pain.

10. Pressing the Juque Point

Location: In the upper abdomen above the front central line, in a notch below the bottom of the sternum.

Method: Use overlapped fingers to press it for about two minutes while bending the body forward.

Effect: Improve allergies.

Tips

The natural process of the cold generally lasts for seven days. Therefore medicine for the cold is usually taken for five to seven days while antibiotics are taken for five days or so. Some patients stop taking medicine at once when the case is alleviated for fear that there will be side effects. This is not advisable. If the medicine is not taken continuously, the remaining virus within the body will revive, which will not only lead to the resistance of the virus against the medicine but also make the complications worse.

So when should one terminate the use of medicine? This should take place after it has been used for the full prescribed course, and when headache, runny nose and cough are completely eliminated and normal temperature returns. The patient should see a doctor at once if the cold continues for seven days or the high fever remains unchanged.

39 | Cough

It is a main symptom of diseases of the respiratory system. Dry cough is marked by the absence of sputum or a little sputum, and it often takes place in the early stage of acute pharyngitis and bronchitis. Acute cough is often due to a foreign body in the bronchus. Chronic cough of a long duration often takes place with chronic bronchitis and TB.

Symptoms

Various types of cough result in different symptoms.

Continuous cough: Generally it is a sign of lung diseases marked by continual severe cough and influence on breathing with flushed neck. Additionally it often causes glottis spasm and produces a sound similar to that of a chicken in addition to retching. Once it starts it will last for two to three months before it stops, and no cough medicine is effective for it.

Wet cough: It is named after the sputum involved with this cough. In the early stage it is a mild dry cough with other symptoms of catching a cold, such as fever, sneezing, runny nose and throat discomfort, before turning into a wet cough with sputum, possibly yellow and thick. It takes place with pneumonia, bronchitis, bronchiectasis, lung abscess and cavitary pulmonary tuberculosis.

Dry cough: It is named after the absence of sputum or only a little sputum when coughing. It takes place with acute pharyngitis, bronchitis, early stage tuberculosis and pleurisy.

Dog-barking cough: It is named as such because the sound of the cough is similar to the barking of a dog. It often takes place in the epiglottis, with throat problems or bronchus under pressure. It is commonly seen in acute child laryngitis among babies from six months to three years old.

Target Acupoints

Shoulder, back and waist: Feishu (BL 13), Fengmen (BL 12).
Chest and abdomen: Tiantu (RN 22), Danzhong (RN 17), Zhongfu (LU 1), Shufu (KI 27), Burong (ST 19).
Arms: Lieque (LU 7), Hegu (LI 4), Yuji (LU 10).

Recommended Massage

1. Pressing and Kneading the Feishu Point
Location: At the point 1.5 cun beside the third thoracic vertebra on the inner side of the scapula.

Method: Sit upright. First place the left palm heel on the Jianjing point on the right side, with the middle fingertip pressing, rubbing and kneading the Feishu point

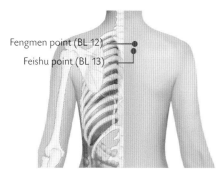

Location of the Fengmen and Feishu points.

Fengmen point (BL 12)
Feishu point (BL 13)

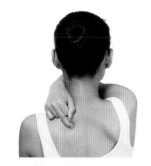

Press and knead the Fengmen point.

on the right side for two minutes. Then place the right palm heel on the Jianjing point on the left side, kneading until the part concerned feels warm as the best effect.

Effect: Treat cold, cough, bronchitis, asthma, spontaneous perspiration, night sweating and back tingling and pain.

2. Pressing and Kneading the Fengmen Point

Location: 1.5 cun below the spinous process of the second thoracic vertebra.

Method: Sit upright. Use the tip of the middle finger of the left hand to press and knead the Fengmen point of the right side. At the same time use the tip of the right middle finger to press and knead the Fengmen point on the left. Continue for two minutes until some tingling and distension are obvious.

Effect: Chiefly serve to cure severe neckback pain, cold and diseases of the respiratory system.

3. Pressing the Tiantu Point

Location: Right in the middle of the cavity above the suprasternal fossa, just between the collarbones.

Method: Sit upright. Use the index fingertip of the left hand to press the Tiantu point, staying still for one minute after moving from the rear margin of the presternum downward. The force of massage is not supposed to affect the breathing of the patient.

Effect: Treat asthma, hiccups, cough, loss of speech, sore throat, thyromegaly, globus hystericus, cough with infection, bronchial asthma, bronchitis, pharyngitis and tonsillitis.

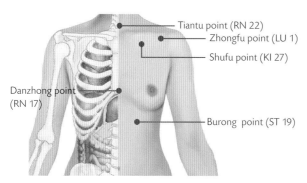

Tiantu point (RN 22)
Zhongfu point (LU 1)
Shufu point (KI 27)
Danzhong point (RN 17)
Burong point (ST 19)

Location of the Tiantu, Zhongfu, Shufu, Danzhong and Burong points.

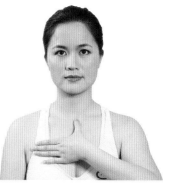

Press the Tiantu point.

---

4. Pressing and Kneading the Shanzhong Point

Location: Directly in the middle of the chest between the nipples.

Method: Sit upright or lie on the back. Use the thenar eminence of the left hand or palm heel to press and knead the point for two minutes, ideally until numbness and distension radiate to the chest. You can also use the thumb pad of the right hand or the thenar eminence to press and knead it for about two minutes, proceeding from light to heavy force.

Effect: Cure difficulty in breathing, cough, chest pain, hyperplasia of the mammary glands, agalactia, palpitation and obesity.

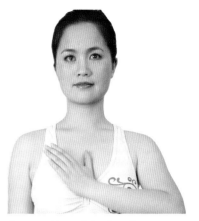

Press and knead the Danzhong point.

5. Pressing and Kneading the Zhongfu Point

Location: At the center of a notch below the S-shaped collarbone in front of the shoulder.

Method: Sit upright or lie on the back. Place the thumb tips on this acupoint on both sides, with the rest of the fingers on the chest. Press forcefully for about 30 seconds continuously, then knead for two minutes.

Effect: Cough will be alleviated with smooth breathing achieved at once. It also serves to treat tracheitis, bronchial asthma, pneumonia, chest pain and shoulder-back pain.

6. Pressing and Kneading the Shufu Point

Location: Two cun horizontally away from the central line on the lower edge of the collarbone.

Method: Sit upright. Use the index or middle finger to press and knead the point on the opposite side about 80 times.

Effect: Chiefly serve to cure cough, asthma, chest pain, vomiting and loss of appetite.

7. Pressing and Kneading the Burong Point

Location: Two cun away from the central line and six cun above the navel.

Method: Sit upright. Use the four fingers together to press and knead the Burong point of the same side for about two minutes in a small circular manner.

Effect: Cure vomiting, gastric diseases, lack of appetite and abdominal distension.

8. Pinching and Kneading the Lieque Point

Location: Take one index finger and put it at the top of the opposite thumb, then slide it in until the tip of the index finger crosses the back of the wrist of the opposite hand. The index finger is now touching the opposite Lieque point.

Method: Sit upright or lie on the back. Use the thumb to forcefully pinch and press the point

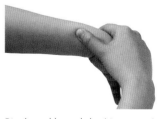

Pinch and knead the Lieque point.

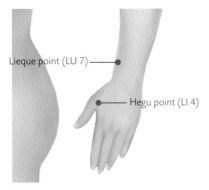

Location of the Liequ and Hegu points.

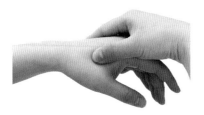

Pinch and knead the Hegu point.

upward for one minute. Then gently knead it for another two minutes, until tingling and distension are felt as the best effect.

Effect: Cure headache, migraine, stiff neck and cough.

9. Pinching and Kneading the Hegu Point

Location: In the highest point on the back of the hand between the thumb base and the base of the index finger (in the webbing between these two fingers).

Method: Use the thumb tip of one hand to pinch the Hegu point on the other hand for about one minute, and continue pinching and kneading for about two minutes, until some tingling and distension are felt as the best effect.

Effect: Treat facioplegia, trigeminal pain, facial paralysis, deviated mouth and eyes (facial paralysis), rhinitis, headache, toothache, acne, visual fatigue, sore throat, tinnitus and hiccups.

10. Pressing and Kneading the Yuji Point

Location: With the palm turned upward, in the depression behind the first metacarpophalangeal joint of the thumb.

Method: Sit upright or lie on the back. Use the thumb to forcefully press the point for 30 seconds. Then continue to press and knead it gently for another two minutes, until tingling and distension are felt as the best effect.

Effect: Treat mastitis, cough, hematemesis, sore throat, fever, tonsillitis, chilblains, wrinkly skin and contraction of the thenar eminence.

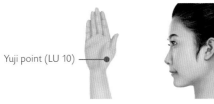

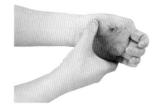

Press and knead the Yuji point.

Tips

Many people believe that they can get through a cough without seeing a doctor. In fact if treatment is not timely and effectively, it will attack frequently, leading to sore throat, hoarseness and chest pain. Therefore attention should be paid to the cough of people who have caught a cold, with appropriate medical treatment.

40 Chronic Bronchial Asthma

It is a common disease, marked by seasonal attack. The reasons include sputum that remains for a long time in lungs, catching a cold, improper diet and bad mood, which results in sputum congestion, blocking the bronchus, and disadvantageous circulation of lung vitality.

Twenty percent of patients with chronic bronchial asthma can trace a family history of the disease. It can happen at any age but generally occurs before age 12. The incidence is roughly the same in male adults and female adults.

Symptoms

Different types of chronic bronchial asthma result in varying symptoms.

Bronchial asthma occurring for over a long time is mostly coupled with emphysema. Patients often feel oppression in the chest with quick breathing and even breathing with wheezing sounds. They often wake up with a start in the middle of the night, coughing with quick breathing and wheezing.

Light asthma: It is marked by oppression in the chest, quick breathing, slight wheezing, less cough and a little sputum. Patients with this kind can engage in work of ordinary types.

Heavy asthma: It often goes together with quite serious emphysema or bronchiectasis, in addition to oppression in the chest, quick breathing, quite obvious wheezing, and frequent cough with a lot of sputum, either white and foamy or as sticky as glue that cannot be coughed out easily. With the sputum coughed out, patients will breathe comfortably, but the case will become worse again when there is an accumulation of sputum. Patients are apt to get infection along with low or high fever caused by acute infection of the respiratory tract. The white sputum will turn into yellow. In general patients of this type have a weak physique coupled with a lack of oxygen. Therefore it is difficult for them to engage in normal work.

Target Acupoints

Head and neck: Renying (ST 9).
Shoulder, back and waist: Dazhui (DU 14), Dingchuan (EX-B 1), Feishu (BL 13), Shenshu (BL 23), Mingmen (DU 4), Gaohuang (BL 43).
Chest and abdomen: Tiantu (RN 22), Danzhong (RN 17), Zhongwan (RN 12).
Legs: Zusanli (ST 36), Fenglong (ST 40), Zutonggu (BL 66).

Recommended Massage

1. Pushing and Pressing the Renying Point
Location: 1.5 cun away from the Adam's apple.

Method: Sit upright or lie on the back while looking up. Use the pad of the thumb and index finger to push and press it up and down.

Effect: It has a very good effect on curing asthma, cough, chronic rheumatic arthritis, high blood pressure, gout, yellowish skin, bronchitis and sore throat, in addition to treating anxiety, angina pectoris, pain of gastric convulsion or gallstones, and various symptoms caused by thyrotoxicosis (hyperthyroidism).

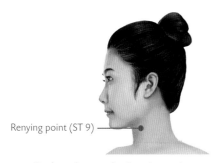

Renying point (ST 9)

Push and press the Renying point.

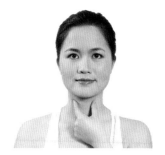

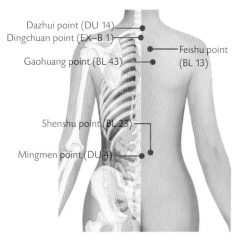

Dazhui point (DU 14)
Dingchuan point (EX–B 1)
Gaohuang point (BL 43)
Feishu point (BL 13)
Shenshu point (BL 23)
Mingmen point (DU 4)

Location of the Dazhui, Dingchuan, Feishu, Gaohuang, Shenshu and Mingmen points.

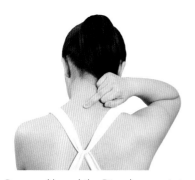

Press and knead the Dingchuan point.

2. Pressing the Dazhui Point

Location: Under the spinous process of the seventh cervical vertebrae.

Method: Sit on a chair. Use the middle finger to press the Dazhui point while extending the elbow and leaning backward.

Effect: An important acupoint for health care, it serves to enhance the ability of preventing diseases, and to treat head-neck pain, neck-shoulder syndrome, cervical spondylosis, fever, cold, asthma, malaria, chronic bronchitis, tuberculosis (TB) and epilepsy as well as cold limbs, shoulder-back cold pain and physical weakness caused by the lack of vital energy.

3. Pressing and Kneading the Dingchuan Point

Location: At the point 0.5 cun away from the spinous process of the seventh cervical vertebra.

Method: Sit upright. Use the middle or index finger of the left hand to press and knead the Dingchuan point. Then use the middle or index finger of the right hand to press and knead the point, two minutes each time, until tingling and distension are obvious in the part concerned as the best effect.

Effect: Cure athsma, cough, pain in the shoulder and back, stiff neck.

4. Pressing the Feishu Point

Location: At the point 1.5 cun beside the third thoracic vertebra on the inner side of the scapula.

Method: Sit upright. First place the left palm heel on the Jianjing point on the right side, with the middle fingertip pressing, rubbing and kneading the Feishu point on the right side for two minutes. Then place the right palm heel on the Jianjing point on the left side, kneading until the part concerned feels hot as the best effect.

Effect: Treat cold, cough, bronchitis, asthma, spontaneous perspiration, night sweating and back tingling and pain.

5. Pressing and Kneading the Gaohuang Point

Location: Three cun away from the spinous process of the fourth cervical vertebra.

Method: Sit upright. Use the four fingers to press and knead the point for about two minutes while using the other hand to hold the elbow, turning the body inward during massage.

Effect: Chiefly serve to cure cough, asthma, TB, forgetfulness and nocturnal emission.

6. Pressing and Kneading the Shenshu Point

Location: 1.5 cun horizontally from the second lumbar spinal process.

Method: Lie on the back or sit upright. Use the two middle fingers to forcefully press and knead the Shenshu point of both sides 30 to 50 times, keeping the thumbs by the ribs. Or, with a clenched fist, use the knuckle of the index finger to press and knead the Shenshu point 30 to 50 times. You might also try using a loose fist to knead and rub 30 to 50 times, until some warmth is felt as the best effect.

Effect: Treat waist tingling and leg pain, lumbar muscle strain, lumbar disc herniation, leg swelling, fatigue all over the body, impotence, nocturnal emission, premature ejaculation and menstrual disorder.

7. Pressing the Mingmen Point

Location: In a cavity below the spinous process of the second cervical vertebra.

Method: Sit upright or lie on the back, with the back straightening up slightly. Use the back of the palm or the knuckles to press the point rhythmically for two minutes with a little heavier force.

Effect: Treat severe waist pain, leg paralysis, menstrual disorder, reddish leucorrhea, dysmenorrhea, amenorrhea and infertility, as well as nocturnal emission, impotence, infertility due to cold sperm, frequent urination, cold pain in the lower abdomen, and diarrhea.

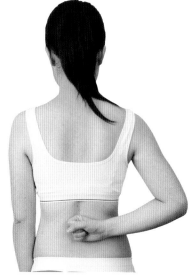

Press the Mingmen point.

8. Pressing the Tiantu Point

Location: Right in the middle of the cavity above the suprasternal fossa, just between the collarbones.

Method: Sit upright. Use the thumb tip of the left hand to press the Tiantu point, staying still for one minute after moving from the rear margin of the presternum downward. The force of massage is not supposed to affect the breathing of the patient.

Effect: Treat asthma, hiccups, cough, loss of speech, sore throat, thyromegaly, globus hystericus, cough with infection, bronchial asthma, bronchitis, pharyngitis and tonsillitis.

9. Pressing and Kneading the Danzhong Point

Location: Directly in the middle of the chest between the nipples.

Method: Sit upright or lie on the back. Use the thumb pad or the thenar eminence of the right hand to press and knead the point for about two minutes, proceeding from light to heavy force.

Effect: It serves to cure difficulty in breathing, fluster, palpitation, cough, chest pain, hyperplasia of mammary glands, breast pain, the lack of human milk and obesity, etc.

10. Pressing the Zhongwan Point

Location: In between the lower part of the sternum and the navel.

Method: Sit upright or lie on the back. Use the middle or index finger to press and knead the point downward for two minutes, until tingling and distension are felt as the best effect.

Effect: Cure low blood pressure, anemia, abdominal distension and pain, acid regurgitation, vomiting and constipation.

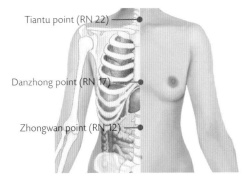
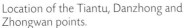

Location of the Tiantu, Danzhong and Zhongwan points.

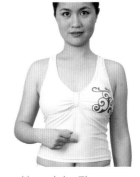

Press and knead the Zhongwan point.

11. Pressing and Kneading the Fenglong Point

Location: Eight cun above the ankle tip.

Method: Sit upright. Use the thumb pad to press and knead the Fenglong points on both sides for two minutes, until tingling and distension are felt as the best effect.

Effect: Chiefly serve to treat mental disorders such as hysteria, insomnia and headache, as well as diseases of the circulatory system, such as high blood pressure, cerebral hemorrhage and the aftereffect of cerebrovascular diseases. It is beneficial for diseases of the respiratory system, such as acute and chronic bronchitis, asthma and pleurisy, as well as diseases of the digestive system, such as hepatitis, appendicitis, and constipation. In addition it can cure urine retention, addiction to smoking, obesity, leg-knee tingling and pain, and shoulder periarthritis.

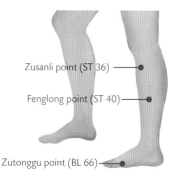

Location of the Zusanli, Fenglong and Zutonggu points.

12. Pressing and Kneading the Zusanli Point

Location: About three cun below the knee on the outer side of the tibia.

Method: Sit upright. Use both thumbs to press the point on both sides, with the four fingers alongside the outer side of the lower leg, pressing and kneading outward 20 to 40 times, until some tingling and distension are felt as the best effect.

Effect: Cure anemia, low blood pressure, diarrhea, abdominal pain, lack of appetite, constipation, vomiting, menopause syndrome and waist-leg pain.

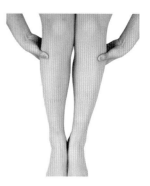

Press and knead the Zusanli point.

13. Pressing and Kneading the Zutonggu Point

Location: Along the outer side of the foot, at the border of the sole (which will be marked by a change to lighter skin in many people), at the far end of the fifth metatarsophalangeal joint.

Method: Sit with crossed legs. Hold one knee while using the thumb to press the Zutonggu point of the same side. Bend the finger joint into a ninety-degree angle to press, rub and knead a small area in a circular manner.

Effect: Chiefly serve to cure headache, stiff neck, dizziness, nose bleeding and epilepsy.

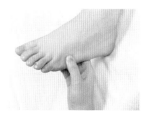

Press and knead the Zutonggu point.

Tips

Dangerous factors for asthma can be due to heredity and the environment. Avoiding unhealthy environmental factors can help prevent asthma.

- Reduce the presence of foreign bodies in the room, such as mold and fungi, and avoid dampness.
- Do not grow plants with flowers.
- Shut doors and windows when there is pollen present.
- Do not keep any pets to prevent asthma due to the fur of pets.
- Eliminate insects as the excrement of some kinds (chiefly cockroaches) can lead to asthma.

41 Lack of Blood Supply to the Brain

A kind of ischemic cerebrovascular disease, it is brainstem ischemia mostly caused by inadequate blood supply to the vertebral artery and basilar artery. This is mostly related to high blood pressure and atherosclerosis as well as the vertebral artery pressed by cervical spine hyperplasia, which requires timely treatment.

Symptoms

Many people, particularly middle-aged and older people, often suffer from dizziness and headache along with agitation, tinnitus, difficulty sleeping with lots of dreams, distraction and forgetfulness. These may be symptoms of inadequate blood supply to the brain, which will first lead to dizziness, nausea and vomiting. Patients avoid moving the head and they may not even dare to open their eyes, which will make dizziness worse. The above-mentioned symptoms will become worse if the patient turns the head sharply or rotates it. When the direction stabilizes, those symptoms will immediately take a turn for the better or disappear.

Target Acupoints

Head and neck: Baihui (DU 20), Taiyang (EX-HN 5), Sishencong (EX-HN 1), Fengchi (GB 20), Tianzhu (BL 10), Touwei (ST 8).
Shoulder, back and waist: Dazhui (DU 14).

Recommended Massage

1. Pinching and Pressing the Baihui Point
Location: At the center of the skull directly on top of the head, over the two ear tips.

Method: Sit upright or lie on the back. Use the middle or index finger to pinch and press the point 20 to 30 times, proceeding from light to heavy force.

Effect: Treat headache caused by high blood pressure, dizziness, panic, forgetfulness, low blood pressure, apoplexy, epilepsy, hysteria, tinnitus and insomnia.

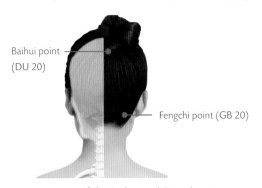

Baihui point (DU 20)

Fengchi point (GB 20)

Location of the Baihui and Fengchi points.

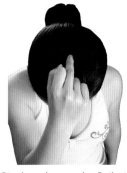

Pinch and press the Baihui point.

2. Pressing and Kneading the Fengchi Point

Location: In the depression on both sides of the large tendon behind the nape of the neck, next to the lower edge of the skull.

Method: Place the thumb pads on the Fengchi point on either side of the head, with the remaining fingers holding the head. Press, rub and knead for two minutes proceeding from light to heavy force until you feel tingling and distension in the related part.

Effect: Treat cold, fever, neck pain, headache, dizziness, and red and swollen eyes with pain.

3. Pressing and Kneading the Touwei Point

Location: Front of the head at the hairline, 0.5 cun from the center line on both sides.

Method: Sit upright. Use the index finger to press and knead the Touwei points of both sides for about two minutes, until tingling and distension are felt, ideally radiating to the entire forehead and both sides.

Effect: Increase longevity, reduce wrinkles, and prevent hair from becoming sparse, split or gray, in addition to curing itchy scalp, migraine, forehead neuralgia, high blood pressure, conjunctivitis and decline of eyesight.

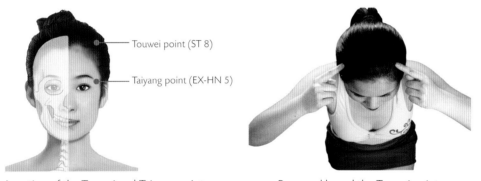

Touwei point (ST 8)

Taiyang point (EX-HN 5)

Location of the Touwei and Taiyang points.   Press and knead the Touwei point.

4. Pressing and Kneading the Taiyang Point

Location: In the depression about one cun behind the space between the outer tip of the brow and outer eye corner.

Method: Sit upright or lie on the back. Use the pad of the index finger to press the Taiyang points on both sides of the head, rubbing and kneading for two minutes until you feel tingling and expansion in the acupoints. If rubbing and kneading of a larger area is required, or you need more force, use the thenar eminences.

Effect: Cure cold, headache, fever, dizziness, and red and swollen eyes with pain.

5. Pressing and Kneading the Sishencong Points

Location: Four points that are one cun away from the Baihui point in each of the four directions.

Method: Sit upright. Use the index and middle fingers of both hands to press and knead the points, two minutes for each of them, until tingling and distension are felt as the best effect.

Effect: Cure neurasthenia, insomnia, dizziness, forgetfulness and deafness.

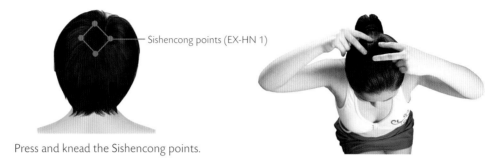

Sishencong points (EX-HN 1)

Press and knead the Sishencong points.

6. Pressing the Tianzhu Point

Location: At the rear of the head, 1.5 cun from the middle line and one cun above the hairline.

Method: Using the thumb, press the Tianzhu point of the same side of the head. As the head turns to the other side, the thumb should press downwards on the Tianzhu point in a slanting manner.

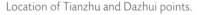

Tianzhu point (BL 10)

Dazhui point (DU 14)

Location of Tianzhu and Dazhui points.

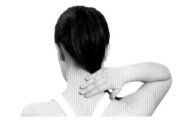

Rubbing the Dazhui point.

Effect: Get rid of cold, tranquilize the spirit, and cure fever, dizziness, neck-shoulder tingling and pain, cervical spondylosis, drowsiness, fatigue, low blood pressure, high blood pressure, drunkenness and car sickness.

7. Rubbing the Dazhui Point

Location: Under the spinous process of the seventh cervical vertebrae.

Method: With four fingers closed and placed on the neck, use the left hand and then the right hand to rub the Dazhui point 30 to 50 times, moving in a slanting way, until some warmth is felt as the best effect.

Effect: Cure cold, fever, stiff neck, severe neck pain, cough and asthma.

Tips

- Eat more fresh vegetables and fruits.
- Exercise moderately, such as walking, 30 to 40 minutes each time for at least five days a week.
- Keep a sound mentality and avoid excitement and overwork.

42 Palpitation and Anxiety

With similar manifestations, both palpitation and anxiety can result in quick heartbeat along with discomfort in the heart and/or stomach. They occur in relation to many kinds of diseases, in association with insomnia, forgetfulness, dizziness and tinnitus. Palpitation can be caused by the abnormality of heartbeat frequency and heart rhythm due to various reasons.

Symptoms

It is chiefly manifested by quick heartbeat and panic. Some people with no medical condition may also experience palpitation or anxiety after athletic activities or excitement.

Target Acupoints

Shoulder, back and waist: Xinshu (BL 15).
Chest and abdomen: Danzhong (RN 17), Wuyi (ST 15).
Arms: Shenmen (HT 7), Neiguan (PC 6).
Legs: Sanyinjiao (SP 6), Yongquan (KI 1).

Recommended Massage

1. Pressing and Kneading the Xinshu Point
Location: Under the fifth thoracic vertebra on the inner side of the scapula, 1.5 cun horizontally away.

Method: Sit upright. Use the tips of both middle fingers to press the Xinshu point of each side respectively for two minutes, ideally until some warmth is felt.

Effect: Cure anxiety and palpitation, shortness of breath, heart pain, cough, hematemesis, chest-back pain, insomnia, forgetfulness, night-sweating, wet dream and epilepsy.

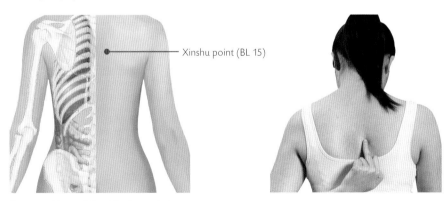

Xinshu point (BL 15)

Press and knead the Xinshu point.

2. Palm Kneading the Danzhong Point

Location: Directly in the middle of the chest between the nipples.

Method: Use the thenar eminence of the left hand or the palm heel against the Danzhong point, kneading it 30 to 40 times. Then use the right hand to knead 30 to 40 times, until distension and numbness radiate to the chest as the best effect.

Effect: Cure difficulty in breathing, cough, chest pain, hyperplasia of the mammary glands, breast pain, agalactia (lactation difficulty), palpitation and obesity.

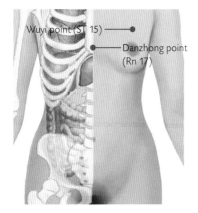

Location of the Wuyi and Danzhong points.

3. Pressing and Kneading the Wuyi Point (on the Left)

Location: At the point directly above the nipple in the second intercostal space.

Method: Sit upright or lie on the back. Use the pad of the middle finger to press and knead the point for about two minutes with moderate force, until tingling and distension are felt as the best effect.

Effect: Cure chest rib pain, breast inflammation, breast distension and pain, hyperplasia of the mammary glands, cough, asthma and vomiting of blood with pus.

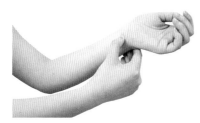

Pinch and press the Shenmen point.

4. Pinching and Pressing the Shenmen Point

Location: On the inner wrist near the small finger when the palm is turned upward.

Method: Use the thumb tip of one hand to pinch and press the point for about one minute and then use the other hand, alternately until tingling and distension are felt as the best effect.

Effect: Treat insomnia, disturbing dreams, anxiety, palpitation, neurasthenia and schizophrenia.

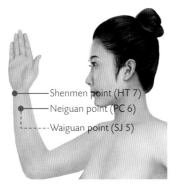

Location of the Shenmen, Neiguan and Waiguan points.

5. Pressing the Neiguan and Waiguan Points

Location: Between the two tendons about two cun above the wrist joint bend.

Method: With the front arm bent halfway, use one thumb tip to press the Neiguan point on the other arm. The index or middle finger should press the Waiguan point, pressing inward 20 to 30 times, until tingling and distension are felt.

Effect: Treat agitation, anxiety, palpitation, angina pectoris, chest distress, chest pain, coronary heart disease, insomnia, gastric and intestinal neurosis.

6. Pressing and Kneading the Sanyinjiao Point

Location: At the rear edge of the shinbone, three cun above the ankle.

Method: Sit upright and place one shin on the opposite thigh. Use the thumb to press, rub and knead the Sanyinjiao point for about two minutes until tingling and distension are felt in the part concerned as the best effect.

Effect: Cure insomnia, high blood pressure, decline of appetite, tension before menstruation, menstrual disorder, dysmenorrhea, impotence and nocturnal emission.

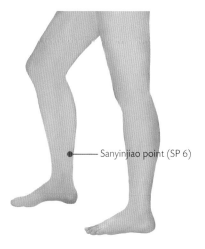

Sanyinjiao point (SP 6)

Location of the Sanyinjiao point.

7. Pushing and Pressing the Yongquan Point

Location: In a depression in the front of the sole of the foot, about one-third of the way down from the toes.

Method: Use the small thenar (hypothenar) eminence of the left hand to forcefully push and press the Yongquan point of the right foot, and use the small thenar eminence of the right hand to push and press the left Yongquan point. Keeping the hand closely attached to the foot, rub back and forth at a high frequency and covering a longer distance, ideally until warmth is felt in the sole.

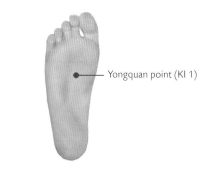

Yongquan point (KI 1)

Location of the Yongquan point.

Effect: Cure foot sole pain and swelling, pale or peeling foot skin, fever, nasal discomfort, allergy, diarrhea, agitation, unconsciousness, insomnia, constipation and difficult urination. Massage can speed up blood circulation of the area and promote metabolism.

Tips

It may be recommended to receive a cardio ECG examination when palpitation occurs frequently. In clinical practice, palpitation is mostly caused by coronary heart disease, which should be considered first when middle-aged and older people suffer from occasional palpitation, chest distress and chest pain.

43 | High Blood Pressure

This is a cardio-vascular disease chiefly marked by the rise of blood pressure of the systemic circulation artery. Blood pressure higher than 140/90 millimeters of mercury can be diagnosed as high blood pressure. As one ages blood pressure will gradually go up correspondingly. High blood pressure is divided into primary and secondary categories. Primary high blood pressure generally refers to a case without other diseases as the cause. Secondary high blood pressure is caused by other kinds of diseases.

Symptoms

According to the degree of urgency of the morbidity, high blood pressure can be divided into chronic and accelerated types with the former being more usual.

Chronic high blood pressure: It is generally marked by dizziness and headache, mostly caused by excitement, fatigue due to excessive work, climatic changes or termination of medicine for lowering blood pressure. The sharp rise of blood pressure may lead to severe headache, blurred vision, nausea, vomiting, convulsion, unconsciousness, transient hemiplegia and loss of speech.

Accelerated high blood pressure: Also called malignant high blood pressure, it suddenly develop from chronic high blood pressure or it may start by itself. It is marked by weakness, thirst, lots of urine, rapid decline of eyesight, and bleeding of the fundus retina, often accompanied by optic disc edema of both sides. In addition there may be the rapid appearance of albumin in the urine, hematuria, renal inadequacy and possibly heart failure, as well as hypertensive crisis and high blood pressure. It usually develops rapidly.

Target Acupoints

Head and neck: Baihui (DU 20), Fengchi (GB 20) and "Reducing-Blood-Pressure-Groove" (auricular acupoint).
Shoulder, back and waist: Ganshu (BL 18).
Arms: Quchi (LI 11).
Legs: Sanyinjiao (SP 6), Taichong (LV 3).

Recommended Massage

1. Rubbing and Kneading the Baihui Point
Location: At the center of the skull directly on top of the head, over the two ear tips.

Method: Sit upright or lie on the back. Use the middle or index finger to pinch and press the point 20 to 30 times, proceeding from light to heavy force.

Effect: Treat headache caused by high blood pressure, dizziness, panic, forgetfulness, low blood pressure, apoplexy, epilepsy, hysteria, tinnitus and insomnia.

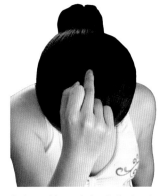

Rub and knead the Baihui point.

2. Smearing the "Reducing-Blood-Pressure-Groove"

Location: In a groove at the back of the ear.

Method: Use the thumb and index finger to pinch the outer ear, with the thumb at the back of the ear and the index finger close to the inside. Keeping the index finger still, use the pad of the thumb to smear from the protruding part of the back of the ear to the earlobe, left and right, 50 times respectively.

Effect: Cure high blood pressure.

3. Pressing and Kneading the Fengchi Point

Location: In the depression on both sides of the large tendon behind the nape of the neck, next to the lower edge of the skull.

Method: Place the thumb pads on the Fengchi point on either side of the head, with the remaining fingers holding the head. Press, rub and knead for two minutes proceeding from light to heavy force until you feel tingling and distension in the related part.

Effect: Cure dizziness caused by high blood pressure, head distension and pain, facial warmth, tinnitus, cold, headache, fever, severe neck pain, and red eyes with swelling and pain.

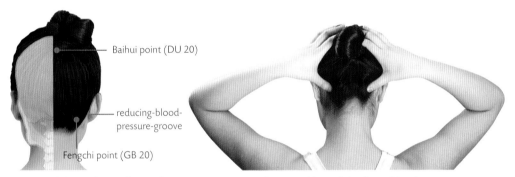

Location of the Baihui and Fengchi points and "reducing-blood-pressure-groove."

Press and knead the Fengchi point.

4. Pressing the Ganshu Point

Location: 1.5 cun away from the ninth thoracic spinal process on the inner side of the scapula.

Method: Sit upright. Use the knuckles of the four fingers to knead the Ganshu point for about two minutes until tingling and distension are felt.

Effect: Treat distension and pain of both sides of the chest, breast pain with swelling, waist-back pain, agitation, irritability, indigestion and aversion to food, neurasthenia, hepatitis, jaundice (icterus), nausea, vomiting, lack of appetite and dizziness.

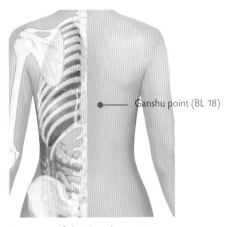

Location of the Ganshu point.

5. Pinching and Pressing the Quchi Point

Location: With the elbow bent halfway, on the outer side of the cubital transverse crease.

Method: Sit upright with the arm half bent. Use the thumb tip to pinch and press the point for one minute and then continue for another two minutes, until tingling and distension are felt as the best effect.

Effect: Prevent and cure cold, high blood pressure, eczema, neurodermatitis, fever, heat-stroke and arm problems.

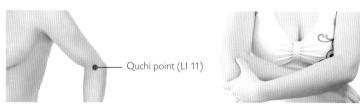

Quchi point (LI 11)

Pinch and press the Quchi point.

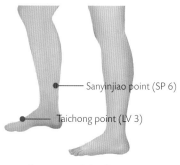

Sanyinjiao point (SP 6)

Taichong point (LV 3)

Location of the Sanyinjiao and Taichong points.

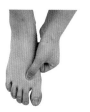

Press and knead the Taichong point.

6. Pressing and Kneading the Sanyinjiao Point

Location: At the rear edge of the shinbone, three cun above the ankle.

Method: Sit upright and place one shin on the opposite thigh. Use the thumb to press, rub and knead the Sanyinjiao point for about two minutes until tingling and distension are felt in the part concerned as the best effect.

Effect: Cure headache caused by high blood pressure, dizziness, short-temper, menstrual disorder, dysmenorrhea, impotence, nocturnal emission and insomnia.

7. Pressing and Kneading the Taichong Point

Location: On the foot in a notch between the first and second metatarsal bones.

Method: Sit upright. Use the thumb or index finger to press the point for 30 seconds and then continue for another two minutes, until tingling and distension are felt as the best effect.

Effect: Cure head distension and pain caused by high blood pressure, dizziness and migraine as well as diseases of gynecology such as menstrual disorder, dysmenorrhea and amenorrhea and breast distension and pain.

Tips

If there are no other reasons for dizziness, headache or the above-mentioned symptoms, then consideration should be given to the possibility of high blood pressure. Once the signs of high blood pressure are discovered, further checkup should be conducted in a timely manner in order to specify diagnosis for early treatment.

44 | Low Blood Pressure

It refers to the condition when the blood pressure of the systemic circulation artery is lower than the normal state. Generally speaking this is determined when the blood pressure of a limb artery of an adult is lower than 90/60 millimeters of mercury.

Symptoms

There are many causes for low blood pressure. Generally speaking it is divided into three categories: primary, orthostatic and symptomatic.

Primary low blood pressure: Patients may be free from symptoms, or suffer from dizziness, seeing stars, forgetfulness, weakness, tinnitus and even unconsciousness.

Orthostatic low blood pressure: There will be the above-mentioned symptoms when patients suddenly stand up from sleeping, sitting and squatting postures, or stand for a long time afterward. These symptoms will be alleviated after returning to the original posture or lying down.

Symptomatic low blood pressure: Patients mostly suffer from some primary disease.

Target Acupoints

Head and neck: Renzhong (DU 26), Baihui (DU 20), Yintang (EX-HN 3), Suliao (DU 25), Tinggong (SI 19).
Shoulder, back and waist: Ganshu (BL 18), Pishu (BL 20), Weishu (BL 21).
Chest and abdomen: Zhongwan (RN 12), Qihai (RN 6).
Arms: Neiguan (PC 6).
Legs: Zusanli (ST 36), Yongquan (KI 1).

Recommended Massage

1. Pinching and Pressing the Baihui Point
Location: At the center of the skull directly on top of the head, over the two ear tips.

Method: Sit upright or lie on the back. Use the middle or index finger to pinch and press the point 20 to 30 times, proceeding from light to heavy force.

Effect: Cure dizziness caused by low blood pressure, visual dizziness, headache, panic, forgetfulness, stroke, tinnitus and insomnia.

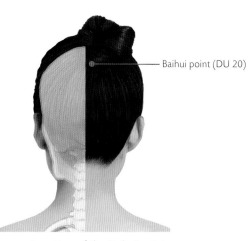

Baihui point (DU 20)

Location of the Baihui point.

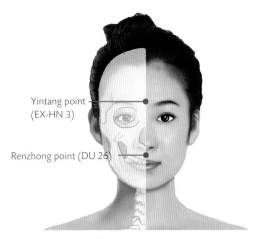

Location of the Yintang and Renzhong points.

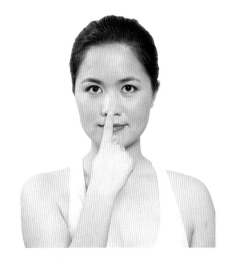

Press the Suliao point.

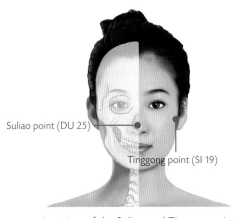

Location of the Suliao and Tinggon points.

2. Pressing and Pinching the Renzhong Point

Location: In the middle of the groove below the nose, between the lip and the nose.

Method: Lie on the back. Use the thumb tip to press and pinch the Renzhong point for one minute with somewhat heavy force, until tingling and distension are felt as the best effect.

Effect: Raise blood pressure, influence breathing and benefit rhythmic respiration, as well as treat unconsciousness, angina, severe waist-back pain and difficulty in breathing.

3. Pushing the Yintang Point

Location: At the central point right between the eyebrows.

Method: Sit upright or lie on the back. Use the pad of the middle finger to push the point up and down. Move first toward the hairline 10 to 20 times, and then down to the nose bridge 10 to 20 times, until some warmth and distension are felt, which can sometimes radiate to the nose.

Effect: Treat cold, vascular headache, frontal sinusitis, supra-orbital neuralgia, acute and chronic rhinitis, nose bleeding, nasal polyp, panasthenia, malaria, nervous vomiting, postpartum anemic fainting, eclampsia, febrile convulsion, convulsion of facial muscles, facioplegia, and acute and chronic conjunctivitis.

4. Pressing the Suliao Point

Location: Right at the center of the nose tip.

Method: Use the index or middle finger to press the point for 30 seconds and then relax for three seconds, repeating 30 times, until some tingling and distension are felt as the best effect.

Effect: Cure acne rosacea, nasal congestion, nose bleeding, runny nose, spasms and unconsciousness.

5. Pressing the Tinggong Point

Location: With the mouth open, in a cavity before the tragus on a line with the earlobe.

Method: Use the radialis of the thumbs to massage the Tinggong points on both sides, up and down 10 to 20 times. Then use the thumb tip to press the Tinggong point for one minute while opening the mouth slightly. There will be slight warmth during massage as well as an alternating feeling of blockage and openness inside the ears that accompanies the pressing. Upon completion there should be an improvement of hearing.

Effect: An acupoint of special curative effect, it serves to cure tinnitus and difficulty hearing, headache, dizziness, decline of eyesight and memory, and trigeminal neuralgia caused by problems with the muscles of the ears and face.

6. Pressing the Ganshu Point

Location: 1.5 cun away from the ninth thoracic spinal process on the inner side of the scapula.

Method: Sit upright. Use the knuckles of the four fingers to knead the Ganshu point for about two minutes until tingling and distension are felt.

Effect: Treat distension and pain of both sides of the chest, breast pain with swelling, waist-back pain, agitation, irritability, indigestion and aversion to food, neurasthenia, hepatitis, jaundice (icterus), nausea, vomiting, lack of appetite and dizziness.

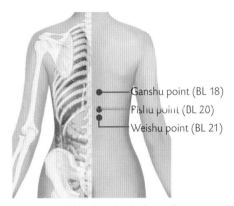

Location of the Ganshu, Pishu and Weishu points.

7. Pressing and Kneading the Weishu Point

Location: About 1.5 cun below the spinous process of the twelfth thoracic vertebra.

Method: Sit or stand. Use the middle fingers to press and knead the Weishu point of both sides (with the thumb against the ribs) forcefully for two minutes. Alternately make a fist and use the protruding index knuckle to press and knead it for two minutes. Or with a loose fist, press and rub the point for two minutes. In all cases some tingling and distension are felt as the best effect.

Effect: Treat all kinds of diseases and symptoms of the digestive system, such as acute gastritis, chronic gastritis, gastroptosis, stomach atony, abdominal distension, abdominal pain, lack of appetite, nausea and vomiting.

8. Pressing and Kneading the Pishu Point

Location: At the point 1.5 cun away horizontally from the eleventh thoracic vertebra.

Method: Sit or stand. Use both middle fingers to press the Pishu point, with the thumb against the ribs, forcefully pressing and kneading for two minutes. Or with a clenched fist, use the index knuckle to press and knead the Pishu point for two minutes. Alternatively you may use a hollow fist to knead and rub it for two minutes, until some tingling and distension are felt.

Effect: Cure nausea, vomiting, abdominal distension, diarrhea, hemafecia (bloody stool) and jaundice.

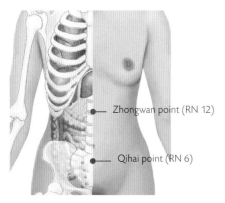

Location of the Zhongwan and Qihai points.

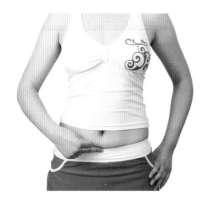

Press and knead the Qihai point.

9. Pressing the Zhongwan Point

Location: In between the lower part of the sternum and the navel.

Method: Sit upright or lie on the back. Use the middle or index finger to press the point downward for two minutes, until some tingling and distension are felt as the best effect.

Effect: Cure low blood pressure, anemia, abdominal distension and pain, diarrhea, acid regurgitation, vomiting and constipation.

10. Pressing and Kneading the Qihai Point

Location: About 1.5 cun below the navel.

Method: Sit upright or lie on the back. Use the index or middle finger to press and knead the point for two minutes, ideally until warmth is felt.

Effect: Cure abdominal pain and distension, constipation or diarrhea, menstrual disorder, dysmenorrhea, amenorrhea, impotence, premature ejaculation and nocturnal emission.

11. Pressing the Neiguan and Waiguan Points

Location: Between the two tendons about two cun above the wrist joint bend.

Method: Bend the forearm halfway. Use the thumb tip of one hand to press the Neiguan point while using the index or middle finger to press the Waiguan point, pressing inward 20 to 30 times.

Effect: Cure agitation, anxiety, palpitation, angina, chest distress, chest pain, coronary heart disease, insomnia, and gastric and intestinal neurosis.

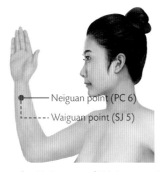

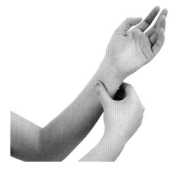

Press the Neiguan and Waiguan points.

12. Pressing and Kneading the Zusanli Point

Location: About three cun below the knee on the outer side of the tibia.

Method: Sit upright. Use both thumbs to press the point on both sides, with the four fingers alongside the outer side of the lower leg, pressing and kneading outward 20 to 40 times, until some tingling and distension are felt as the best effect.

Effect: Treat diarrhea, abdominal pain and distension, lack of appetite, constipation, hiccups, vomiting, anemia, low blood pressure, menopause syndrome and waist-leg pain.

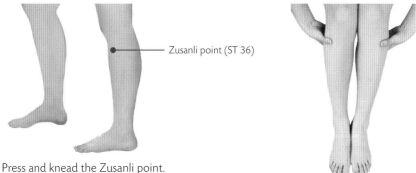

Zusanli point (ST 36)

Press and knead the Zusanli point.

13. Pushing and Pressing the Yongquan Point

Location: In a depression in the front of the sole of the foot, about one-third of the way down from the toes.

Method: Sit while stretching one leg straight, with the other leg placed on the knee of the stretched leg. Use one hand to hold the foot back while using the thumb of the other hand to press and knead the point in a small area vertically for two minutes.

Effect: Treat pain and distension of the sole of the foot, pale or peeling foot skin, fever, nasal discomfort and allergy, diarrhea, agitation, dizziness, insomnia, constipation and difficult urination. Some massage serves to speed up blood circulation in the foot and promote metabolism.

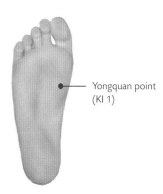

Yongquan point (KI 1)

Location of the Yongquan point.

> **Tips**
> - Keep a sound attitude and do moderate exercise to reduce the morbidity of orthostatic low blood pressure.
> - Avoid fatigue from excessive work because extreme fatigue will further lower blood pressure.
> - Adjust diet and do not eat too much at each meal.
> - Drink some light salty water or eat some slightly salty food every day to increase the amount of fluid and raise blood pressure.

45 | Neurasthenia

This is a state in which the patient exhausts the brain too much for a long time, leading to the decline of mental activities. At present most experts believe that the mental factor is the main reason for neurasthenia. Continuous tension or internal conflict over a long duration will intensify and prolong nerve activities, exceeding the tolerance of the nervous system and therefore leading to neurasthenia.

Symptoms

Neurasthenia is marked by easy mental fatigue, dullness of the mind, difficulty in concentrating, decline of memory, inability to maintain work and study, more recollection and association, lack of control, aversion to sound and light, agitation and easy irritation.

It can also be marked by malfunction of the automatic nerve system manifesting as anxiety, oppression in the chest, difficulty breathing, shortness of breath, agitation, low spirits, and headache caused by tension. In terms of sleep, the patient finds it difficult to fall asleep, wakes up easily during the night and can rarely fall asleep again. One may still feel weak after staying in bed for a long time, and may also feel distended in the head and dizzy.

Target Acupoints

Head and neck: Baihui (DU 20), Taiyang (EX-HN 5), Yintang (EX-HN 3), Sishencong (EX-HN 1).
Shoulder, back and waist: Xinshu (BL 15), Pishu (BL 20), Ganshu (BL 18), Weishu (BL 21), Gaohuang (BL 43).
Arms: Neiguan (PC 6), Shenmen (HT 7).
Legs: Zusanli (ST 36), Yongquan (KI 1).

Recommended Massage

1. Pressing and Kneading the Baihui Point
Location: At the center of the skull directly on top of the head, over the two ear tips.

Method: Sit upright or lie on the back. Use the middle or index finger to press and knead the point for two minutes, proceeding from light to heavy force, until some tingling and distension are felt as the best effect.

Effect: Treat headache caused by high blood pressure, dizziness, panic, forgetfulness, apoplexy, epilepsy, hysteria, tinnitus and insomnia.

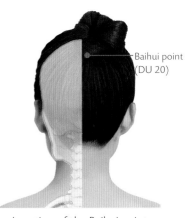

Baihui point (DU 20)

Location of the Baihui point.

2. Pressing and Kneading the Taiyang Point

Location: In the depression about one cun behind the space between the outer tip of the brow and outer eye corner.

Method: Sit upright or lie on the back. Use the pad of the index finger to press the Taiyang points on both sides of the head, rubbing and kneading for two minutes until you feel tingling and expansion in the acupoints. If rubbing and kneading of a larger area is required, or you need more force, use the thenar eminences.

Effect: Cure cold, headache, fever, dizziness, and red and swollen eyes with pain.

3. Pushing the Yintang Point

Location: At the central point right between the eyebrows.

Method: Sit upright or lie on the back. Use the pad of the index finger to push the point up and down. Move first toward the hairline 10 to 20 times, and then down to the nose bridge 10 to 20 times, until some warmth and distension are felt, which can sometimes radiate to the nose.

Effect: Treat cold, vascular headache, frontal sinusitis, supra-orbital neuralgia, rhinitis, nose bleeding, nasal polyp, high blood pressure, neurasthenia, malaria, nervous vomiting, postpartum anemic fainting, febrile convulsion, convulsion of the facial muscles, face-eye paralysis and conjunctivitis.

4. Pressing the Sishencong Points

Location: Four points that are one cun away from the Baihui point in each of the four directions.

Method: Sit upright. Use the index and middle fingers of both hands to press and knead the points, two minutes for each of them, until tingling and distension are felt as the best effect.

Effect: Cure neurasthenia, insomnia, dizziness, forgetfulness and deafness.

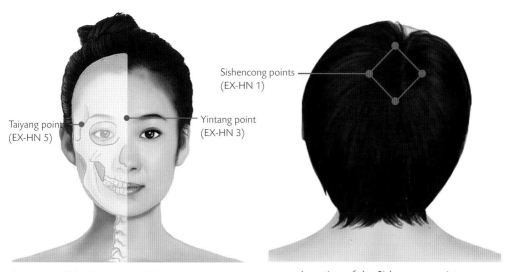

Location of the Taiyang and Yintang points.

Location of the Sishencong points.

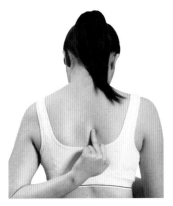

Press and knead the Xinshu point.

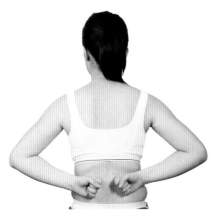

Press and knead the Pishu point.

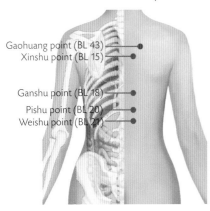

Gaohuang point (BL 43)
Xinshu point (BL 15)

Ganshu point (BL 18)
Pishu point (BL 20)
Weishu point (BL 21)

Location of the Gaohuang, Xinshu, Ganshu, Pishu and Weishu points.

5. Pressing and Kneading the Xinshu Point
Location: Under the fifth thoracic vertebra on the inner side of the scapula, 1.5 cun horizontally away.

Method: Sit on a chair. Use the middle finger to press and knead the Xinshu point for about two minutes, until tingling and distension are felt.

Effect: Treat agitation, palpitation, difficulty breathing, heart pain, cough, hematemesis, chest-back pain, insomnia, forgetfulness, night sweating, wet dream and epilepsy.

6. Pressing and Kneading the Pishu Point
Location: At the point 1.5 cun away horizontally from the eleventh thoracic vertebra.

Method: Sit or stand. Use both middle fingers to press the Pishu point, with the thumb against the ribs, forcefully pressing and kneading for two minutes. Or with a clenched fist, use the index knuckle to press and knead the Pishu point for two minutes. Alternatively you may use a hollow fist to knead and rub it for two minutes, until some tingling and distension are felt.

Effect: Cure nausea, vomiting, abdominal distension, diarrhea, hemafecia (bloody stool) and jaundice.

7. Pressing the Ganshu Point
Location: 1.5 cun away from the ninth thoracic spinal process on the inner side of the scapula.

Method: Sit upright. Use the knuckles of the four fingers to knead the Ganshu point for about two minutes until tingling and distension are felt.

Effect: Treat distension and pain of both sides of the chest, breast pain with swelling, waist-back pain, agitation, irritability, indigestion and aversion to food, neurasthenia, hepatitis, jaundice (icterus), nausea, vomiting, lack of appetite and dizziness.

8. Pressing and Kneading the Weishu Point
Location: About 1.5 cun below the spinous process of the twelfth thoracic vertebra.

Method: Sit or stand. Use the middle fingers to press and knead the Weishu point of both sides (with the thumb against the ribs) forcefully for two minutes.

Alternately make a fist and use the protruding index knuckle to press and knead it for two minutes. Or with a loose fist, press and rub the point for two minutes. In all cases some tingling and distension are felt as the best effect.

Effect: Treat all kinds of diseases and symptoms of the digestive system, such as acute gastritis, chronic gastritis, gastroptosis, stomach atony, abdominal distension, abdominal pain, lack of appetite, nausea and vomiting.

9. Pressing and Kneading the Gaohuang Point
Location: Three cun away from the spinous process of the fourth cervical vertebra.

Method: Sit upright. Use the four fingers to press and knead the point for about two minutes while using the other hand to hold the elbow, turning the body inward during massage.

Effect: Chiefly serve to cure cough, asthma, TB, forgetfulness and nocturnal emission.

10. Pressing the Neiguan and Waiguan Points
Location: Between the two tendons about two cun above the wrist joint bend.

Method: Bend the forearm halfway. Use the thumb tip of one hand to press the Neiguan point while using the index or middle finger to press the Waiguan point, pressing inward 20 to 30 times.

Effect: Cure agitation, anxiety, palpitation, angina, chest distress, chest pain, coronary heart disease, insomnia, and gastric and intestinal neurosis.

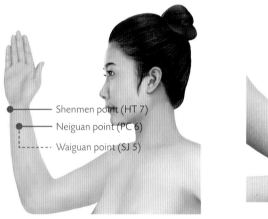

Shenmen point (HT 7)
Neiguan point (PC 6)
Waiguan point (SJ 5)

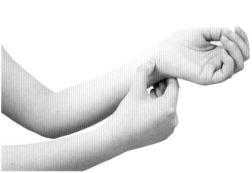

Location of the Shenmen, Neiguan and Waiguan points.   Pinch and press the Shenmen point.

11. Pinching and Pressing the Shenmen Point
Location: On the inner wrist near the small finger when the palm is turned upward.

Method: Use the thumb tip of one hand to pinch and press the point for about one minute and then use the other hand, alternately until tingling and distension are felt as the best effect.

Effect: Treat insomnia, disturbing dreams, anxiety, palpitation, neurasthenia and schizophrenia.

12. Pressing and Kneading the Zusanli Point

Location: About three cun below the knee on the outer side of the tibia.

Method: Sit upright. Use both thumbs to press the point on both sides, with the four fingers alongside the outer side of the lower leg, pressing and kneading outward 20 to 40 times, until some tingling and distension are felt as the best effect.

Effect: Treat diarrhea, abdominal pain and distension, lack of appetite, constipation, hiccups, vomiting, anemia, low blood pressure, menopause syndrome and waist-leg pain.

13. Pushing and Pressing the Yongquan Point

Location: In a depression in the front of the sole of the foot, about one-third of the way down from the toes.

Method: Use the small thenar (hypothenar) eminence of the left hand to forcefully push and press the Yongquan point of the right foot, and use the small thenar eminence of the right hand to push and press the left Yongquan point. Keeping the hand closely attached to the foot, rub back and forth at a high frequency and covering a longer distance, ideally until warmth is felt in the sole.

Effect: Cure foot sole pain and swelling, pale or peeling foot skin, fever, nasal discomfort, allergy, diarrhea, agitation, unconsciousness, insomnia, constipation and difficult urination. Massage can speed up blood circulation of the area and promote metabolism.

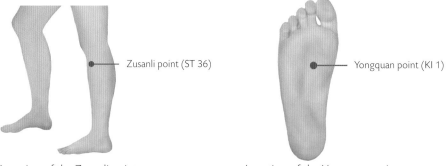

Zusanli point (ST 36)   Yongquan point (KI 1)

Location of the Zusanli point.   Location of the Yongquan point.

Tips
- Patients are advised to take a long walk, which helps to adjust the stimulation of the cerebral cortex, reduce the imbalance of vascular activities, shift attention, and lift the mood. It is important to exercise at the appropriate level: It is suitable for the weak to practice qigong and self-massage. People of average fitness are advised to do exercise for half an hour or one hour. Fitter people can exercise for one to two hours, as well as hike a short distance or take a trip.
- Lots of sweat, excitement or insomnia after exercise indicates excessive volume of exercise, hence requiring the reduction of it.

46 | Insomnia

It may encompass abnormal sleep, difficulty in falling asleep and/or staying asleep, light sleep, frequent dreams and early awakening.

As shown by data from the World Health Organization (WHO), nearly one-quarter of people suffer from insomnia around the world. Among professional women, as high as 80 percent are subject to non-optimal sleep. The relationship between sleep and health is drawing increasing attention.

Symptoms

Medically, insomnia is divided into three kinds: transient insomnia, usually lasting for several days; short-term insomnia, usually lasting for two to three weeks; and long-term chronic insomnia, lasting for over one month. Insomnia lasting for a very long time will not only affect normal work and life, but also influence health.

Target Acupoints

Head, face and neck: Yintang (EX-HN 3), Taiyang (EX-HN 5), Sishencong (EX-HN 1), Anmian (EX-HN 22).
Shoulder, back and waist: Xinshu (BL 15), Weishu (BL 21), Ganshu (BL 18), Pishu (BL 20).
Arms: Shenmen (HT 7).
Legs: Sanyinjiao (SP 6), Yongquan (KI 1).

Recommended Massage

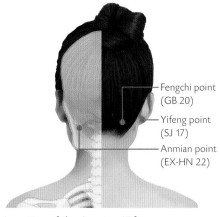

Fengchi point (GB 20)

Yifeng point (SJ 17)

Anmian point (EX-HN 22)

Location of the Anmian, Yifeng and Fengchi points.

1. Pressing and Kneading the Anmian Point

Location: Approximately halfway between the Yifeng point and Fengchi point.

Method: Sit upright, relax the whole body, breathe deeply three times and keep breathing evenly. Use two thumbs to gently press and knead the point for two minutes, until some tingling and distension are felt as the best effect.

Effect: Cure insomnia, anxiety, headache, agitation, dizziness, tinnitus and high blood pressure.

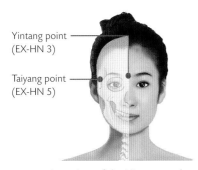

Yintang point
(EX-HN 3)

Taiyang point
(EX-HN 5)

Location of the Yintang and
Taiyang points.

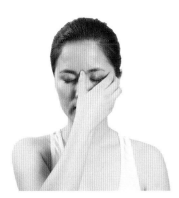

Push and massage
the Yintang point.

2. Pressing and Kneading the Taiyang Point

Location: In the depression about one cun behind the space between the outer tip of the brow and outer eye corner.

Method: Sit upright or lie on the back. Use the pad of the index finger to press the Taiyang points on both sides of the head, rubbing and kneading for two minutes until you feel tingling and expansion in the acupoints. If rubbing and kneading of a larger area is required, or you need more force, use the thenar eminences.

Effect: Cure cold, headache, fever, dizziness, and red and swollen eyes with pain.

3. Pushing and Massaging the Yintang Point

Location: At the central point right between the eyebrows.

Method: Sit upright or lie on the back. Use the thumb to push the point, with the four fingers against the exterior of the eyes. Use the pad of the thumb to push to the hairline, repeating 20 to 30 times.

Effect: Treat cold, vascular headache, frontal sinusitis, supra-orbital neuralgia, rhinitis, nasal polyp, high blood pressure, neurasthenia, malaria, nervous vomiting, postpartum anemic fainting, febrile convulsion, convulsion of the facial muscles, face-eye paralysis and conjunctivitis.

4. Pressing and Kneading the Sishencong Points

Location: Four points that are one cun away from the Baihui point in each of the four directions.

Method: Sit upright. Use the index and middle fingers of both hands to press and knead the points, two minutes for each of them, until tingling and distension are felt as the best effect.

Effect: Cure neurasthenia, insomnia, dizziness, forgetfulness and deafness.

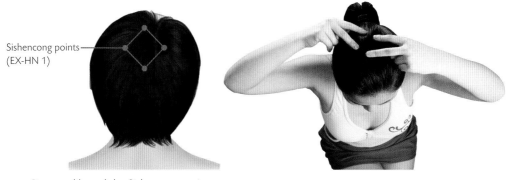

Sishencong points
(EX-HN 1)

Press and knead the Sishencong points.

5. Pressing and Kneading the Weishu Point

Location: About 1.5 cun below the spinous process of the twelfth thoracic vertebra.

Method: Sit or stand. Use the middle fingers to press and knead the Weishu point of both sides (with the thumb against the ribs) forcefully for two minutes. Alternately make a fist and use the protruding index knuckle to press and knead it for two minutes. Or with a loose fist, press and rub the point for two minutes. In all cases some tingling and distension are felt as the best effect.

Effect: Treat all kinds of diseases and symptoms of the digestive system, such as acute gastritis, chronic gastritis, gastroptosis, stomach atony, abdominal distension, abdominal pain, lack of appetite, nausea and vomiting.

6. Pressing and Kneading the Xinshu Point

Location: Under the fifth thoracic vertebra on the inner side of the scapula, 1.5 cun horizontally away.

Method: Sit on a chair. Use the middle finger to press and knead the Xinshu point for about two minutes, until tingling and distension are felt.

Effect: Treat agitation, palpitation, difficulty breathing, heart pain, cough, hematemesis, chest-back pain, insomnia, forgetfulness, night sweating, wet dream and epilepsy.

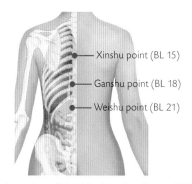
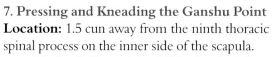

Location of the Xinshu, Ganshu and Weishu points.

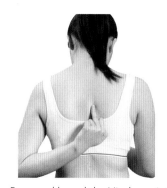

Press and knead the Xinshu point.

7. Pressing and Kneading the Ganshu Point

Location: 1.5 cun away from the ninth thoracic spinal process on the inner side of the scapula.

Method: Sit upright. With clenched fists, use the knuckle of the middle finger to press and knead the point for two minutes, until some tingling and distension are felt as the best effect.

Effect: Cure rib distension during menstruation, breast distension and pain, waist-back pain, easy agitation and anger, aversion to oily food, neurasthenia, hepatitis, jaundice, insomnia, nausea, vomiting, lack of appetite and dizziness.

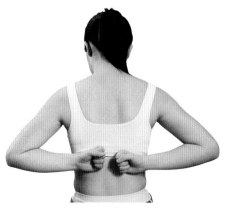

Press and knead the Ganshu point.

8. Pressing and Kneading the Pishu Point

Location: At the point 1.5 cun away horizontally from the eleventh thoracic vertebra.

Method: Sit or stand. Use both middle fingers to press the Pishu point, with the thumb against the ribs, forcefully pressing and kneading for two minutes. Or with a clenched fist, use the index knuckle to press and knead the Pishu point for two minutes. Alternatively you may use a hollow fist to knead and rub it for two minutes, until some tingling and distension are felt.

Effect: Cure nausea, vomiting, abdominal distension, diarrhea, hemafecia (bloody stool) and jaundice.

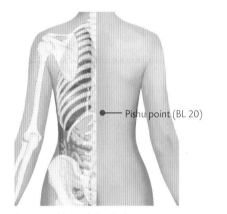
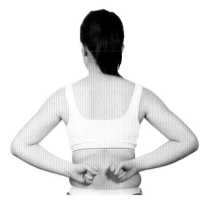

Press and knead the Pishu point.

9. Pressing the Shenmen Point

Location: On the inner wrist near the small finger when the palm is turned upward.

Method: Use the thumb tip of one hand to press the point for about one minute. Then change to press with the other hand, alternating, until some tingling and distension are felt as the best effect.

Effect: Treat insomnia, disordered dreaming, neurasthenia, anxiety and schizophrenia.

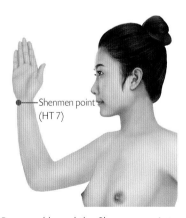
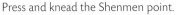
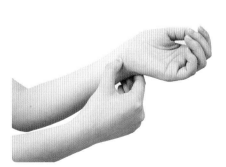

Press and knead the Shenmen point.

10. Pressing and Kneading the Sanyinjiao Point

Location: At the rear edge of the shinbone, three cun above the ankle.

Method: Sit upright and place one shin on the opposite thigh. Use the thumb to press, rub and knead the Sanyinjiao point for about two minutes until tingling and distension are felt in the part concerned as the best effect.

Effect: Cure insomnia, high blood pressure, decline of appetite, tension before menstruation, menstrual disorder, dysmenorrhea, impotence and nocturnal emission.

11. Pushing and Pressing the Yongquan Point

Location: In a depression in the front of the sole of the foot, about one-third of the way down from the toes.

Method: Use the small thenar (hypothenar) eminence of the left hand to forcefully push and press the Yongquan point of the right foot, and use the small thenar eminence of the right hand to push and press the left Yongquan point. Keeping the hand closely attached to the foot, rub back and forth at a high frequency and covering a longer distance, ideally until warmth is felt in the sole.

Effect: Cure foot sole pain and swelling, pale or peeling foot skin, fever, nasal discomfort, allergy, diarrhea, agitation, unconsciousness, insomnia, constipation and difficult urination. Massage can speed up blood circulation of the area and promote metabolism.

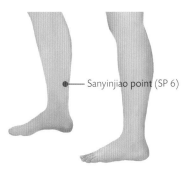

Location of the Sanyinjiao point.

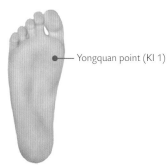

Location of the Yongquan point.

Tips

- Keep an optimistic and contented state of mind.
- Live a life of regular rules and maintain a normal schedule for going to sleep and waking up.
- Exercise moderately in the day time.
- Try not to read, watch television or work in bed before going to sleep.
- Treatment is required as soon as possible if one suffers from quite serious insomnia. Also one should take sleeping pills in a moderate amount for a short time, or anti-agitation or anti-depression medication in a small dosage, under the guidance of the doctor.

47 | Kidney Deficiency and Presenility

In TCM "kidney deficiency" does not refer only to problems with the kidney. It encompasses many kinds of diseases of the urinary, reproductive, endocrine, nervous, digestive, vascular and respiratory systems. Presenility, which refers to a person who becomes old earlier than people of normal health, is associated with kidney deficiency.

Symptoms

It is marked by insomnia, difficulty in concentrating the mind, heat all over the body or unusual fear of the cold, weakness in the waist and legs, and palpebral edema.

Target Acupoints

Head and the neck: Sishencong (EX-HN 1).
Shoulder, back and waist: Ganshu (BL 18), Shenshu (BL 23), Yaoyangguan (DU 3), Mingmen (DU 4).
Chest and abdomen: Qihai (RN 6), Shenque (RN 8), Guanyuan (RN 4).
Legs: Zhaohai (KI 6), Taixi (KI 3), Yongquan (KI 1).

Recommended Massage

1. Pressing the Sishencong Points

Location: Four points that are one cun away from the Baihui point in each of the four directions.

Method: Sit upright. Use the index and middle fingers of both hands to press and knead the points, two minutes for each of them, until tingling and distension are felt as the best effect.

Effect: Cure neurasthenia, insomnia, dizziness, forgetfulness and deafness.

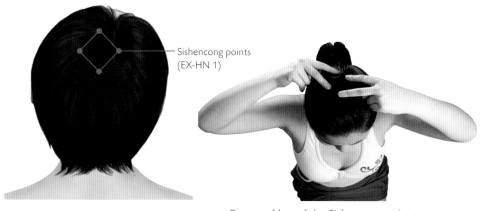

Sishencong points
(EX-HN 1)

Press and knead the Sishencong points.

2. Pressing the Ganshu Point

Location: 1.5 cun away from the ninth thoracic spinal process on the inner side of the scapula.

Method: Sit upright. Use the knuckles of the four fingers to knead the Ganshu point for about two minutes until tingling and distension are felt.

Effect: Treat distension and pain of both sides of the chest, breast pain with swelling, waist-back pain, agitation, irritability, indigestion and aversion to food, neurasthenia, hepatitis, jaundice (icterus), nausea, vomiting, lack of appetite and dizziness.

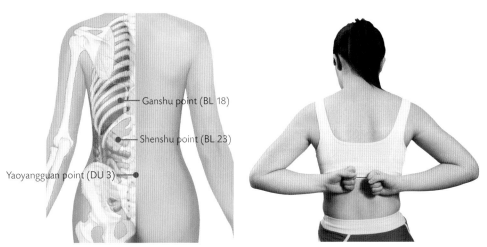

Ganshu point (BL 18)

Shenshu point (BL 23)

Yaoyangguan point (DU 3)

Location of the Ganshu, Shenshu and Yaoyangguan points.

Press the Ganshu point.

3. Pressing and Kneading the Shenshu Point

Location: 1.5 cun horizontally from the second lumbar spinal process.

Method: Lie on the back or sit upright. Use the two middle fingers to forcefully press and knead the Shenshu point of both sides 30 to 50 times, keeping the thumbs by the ribs. Or, with a clenched fist, use the knuckle of the index finger to press and knead the Shenshu point 30 to 50 times. You might also try using a loose fist to knead and rub 30 to 50 times, until some warmth is felt as the best effect.

Effect: Treat waist tingling and leg pain, lumbar muscle strain, lumbar disc herniation, leg swelling, fatigue all over the body, impotence, nocturnal emission, premature ejaculation and menstrual disorder.

4. Pressing the Yaoyangguan Point

Location: In a cavity below the fourth lumbar vertebra.

Method: While standing use the index and middle finger to press the point for two minutes.

Effect: It is very effective in curing cold feeling in the waist. In addition, together with related acupoints of the Governor Meridian, it can cure mental diseases, heat-based diseases and diseases in the waist, back, head and neck as well as corresponding diseases of the inner organs.

5. Pressing the Mingmen Point

Location: In a cavity below the spinous process of the second cervical vertebra.

Method: Sit upright or lie on the back, with the back straightening up slightly. Use the back of the palm or the knuckles to press the point rhythmically for two minutes with a little heavier force.

Effect: Cure severe waist pain, leg paralysis, menstrual disorder, reddish leucorrhea, dysmenorrhea, amenorrhea, infertility, nocturnal emission, impotence, infertility due to cold sperm, frequent urination, cold feeling and pain in lower abdomen, and diarrhea.

6. Pressing and Kneading the Qihai Point

Location: About 1.5 cun below the navel.

Method: Use the tips of the index or middle finger to press and knead the point for two minutes, until warmth is felt as the best effect.

Effect: Cure abdominal pain and distension, constipation or diarrhea, menstrual disorder, dysmenorrhea, amenorrhea, impotence, premature ejaculation and nocturnal emission.

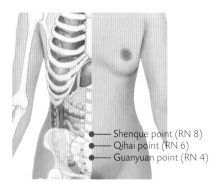 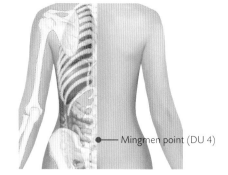

Location of the Shenque, Qihai and Guanyuan points.

7. Massaging the Shenque Point

Location: At the center of the navel.

Method: Use the right palm to massage around the navel gently and slowly, for two to three minutes in a revolving manner, until warmth is felt in the abdomen. It is better to do it one hour after eating.

Effect: Cure cold and pain around the navel, dysmenorrhea, infertility, cold limbs, diarrhea or constipation, and aconuresis (urinary incontinence).

8. Pressing and Kneading the Guanyuan Point

Location: About three cun below the navel.

Method: Sit upright or lie on the back. First use the index or middle finger to press the point for 30 seconds. Then continue to press and knead it for another two minutes, until some tingling and distension are felt as the best effect.

Effect: Cure abdominal pain and distension, menstrual disorder, dysmenorrhea, amenorrhea, nocturnal emission and impotence.

9. Pressing and Kneading the Zhaohai Point

Location: In a cavity below the protruding point in the interior of the ankle.

Method: Sit upright. Use the thumb to press and knead for two minutes, until some tingling and distension are felt as the best effect.

Effect: Treat interior pain after ankle sprain, dry throat, insomnia, addiction to sleep, panic, red eyes with swelling and pain, menstrual disorder, dysmenorrhea, reddish leucorrhea, uterus prolapse, genital itch, hernia, frequent urination and dermatophytosis.

10. Pressing and Kneading the Taixi Point

Location: In a cavity between the medial malleolus and Achilles tendon.

Method: Sit upright. Use the thumb to press and knead the Taixi point for two to three minutes until some tingling and distension are felt. This massage is prohibited during pregnancy.

Effect: Chiefly serve to cure headache, dizzy vision, stiff neck, waist tingling, tinnitus, sore throat, insomnia, frequent urination, bed-wetting, menstrual disorder, ankle swelling and pain, ankle sprain, asthma, nephritis and cystitis.

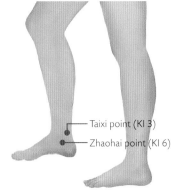

Taixi point (KI 3)
Zhaohai point (KI 6)

Location of the Taixi and Zhaohai points.

11. Pushing and Pressing the Yongquan Point

Location: In a depression in the front of the sole of the foot, about one-third of the way down from the toes.

Method: Use the small thenar (hypothenar) eminence of the left hand to forcefully push and press the Yongquan point of the right foot, and use the small thenar eminence of the right hand to push and press the left Yongquan point. Keeping the hand closely attached to the foot, rub back and forth at a high frequency and covering a longer distance, ideally until warmth is felt in the sole.

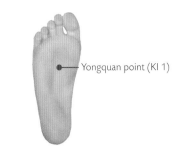

Yongquan point (KI 1)

Location of the Yongquan point.

Effect: Cure foot sole pain and swelling, pale or peeling foot skin, fever, nasal discomfort, allergy, diarrhea, agitation, unconsciousness, insomnia, constipation and difficult urination. Massage can speed up blood circulation of the area and promote metabolism.

Tips

- Do more exercise of the waist.
- Increased massage at the center of the feet serves to prevent presenility, in addition to soothing the liver, brightening eyesight, clearing the throat, calming the heart, promoting sleep and increasing appetite.

48 | Diabetes

It is a syndrome of a series of metabolic disorders of glucose, protein, fat, water and electrolytes caused by the decline of pancreatic function and resistance of insulin due to the impact of hereditary and external factors.

Symptoms

In clinical practice it is chiefly marked by hyperglycemia. Its typical manifestation is described, as translated from the Chinese phrase, as: "three excessiveness and one deficiency." This means there is more urine, more desire to drink, more desire of eating food, and emaciation.

- More urine: There is an increase in the frequency of urinating (i.e. more than 20 times within 24 hours) along with an increase of the amount of urine. Urine appears foamy, while the urine stains look white and sticky.
- Drinking more: With more urine, the amount of water in the body diminishes, resulting in the desire to drink due to stimulation of the thirst center in the brain.
- Eating more: Blood glucose cannot be utilized since it cannot enter cells, stimulating the hunger center in the brain to bring about the desire for more food. There is no sense of fullness after the meal, leading to obvious increase of the frequency of eating and the amount of food eaten.
- Emaciation: Rapid reduction of weight is caused by the decrease of glucose utilization, increase of fat lipolysis, inadequate protein synthesis and acceleration of its decomposition. Excess urination will aggravate emaciation because of the loss of water in the body.

Target Acupoints

Shoulder, back and waist: Yishu (EX-B3), Weishu (BL 21), Pishu (BL 20), Ganshu (BL 18), Shenshu (BL 23), Yishe (BL 49), Sanjiaoshu (BL 22).
Chest and abdomen: Zhongwan (RN 12), Daju (ST 27), Qihai (RN 6).
Legs: Zusanli (ST 36), Yongquan (KI 1), Sanyinjiao (SP 6), Yanglingquan (GB 34).

Recommended Massage

1. Pressing and Kneading the Yishu Point
Location: At the point 1.5 cun away from the spinous process of the eighth thoracic vertebra.

    Method: With fists clenched, use the knuckle of the middle finger to press and knead the point for two minutes, until some tingling and distension are felt as the best effect.

    Effect: Chiefly serve to treat acute and chronic gastritis, gastric ulcer, duodenal ulcer, gastric neurosis, acute and chronic pancreatitis, nervous vomiting, diaphragm spasm, bronchitis, pleurisy, intercostal nerve pain, shingles, diabetes and chronic pharyngitis.

2. Pressing and Kneading the Weishu Point

Location: About 1.5 cun below the spinous process of the twelfth thoracic vertebra.

Method: Sit or stand. Use the two middle fingers to press and knead the Weishu point of both sides forcefully for 30 to 50 times. Alternately make a fist and use the protruding index knuckle to press and knead it for 30 to 50 times. Or with a loose fist, press and rub the point for 30 to 50 times. In all cases some tingling and distension are felt as the best effect.

Effect: Treat all kinds of diseases and symptoms of the digestive system, such as acute gastritis, chronic gastritis, gastroptosis, stomach atony, abdominal distension, abdominal pain, lack of appetite, nausea and vomiting.

3.Pressing and Kneading the Pishu Point

Location: At the point 1.5 cun away horizontally from the eleventh thoracic vertebra.

Method: Sit or stand. Use two middle fingers to forcefully press and knead the Pishu points on both sides 30 to 50 times, with thumbs grasping the ribs. You may also make a fist and use the index knuckle to press and knead 30 to 50 times. Or with hollow fists, knead and rub 30 to 50 times, ideally until some warmth is felt.

Effect: Treat diseases of the spleen, stomach and intestines such as stomachalgia, abdominal distension, diarrhea, vomiting, dysentery, hemafecia and jaundice.

4. Pressing and Kneading the Ganshu Point

Location: 1.5 cun away from the ninth thoracic spinal process on the inner side of the scapula.

Method: Sit upright. Use the knuckles of the four fingers to knead the Ganshu point for about two minutes until tingling and distension are felt.

Effect: Treat distension and pain of both sides of the chest, breast pain with swelling, waist-back pain, agitation, irritability, indigestion and aversion to food, neurasthenia, hepatitis, jaundice (icterus), nausea, vomiting, lack of appetite and dizziness.

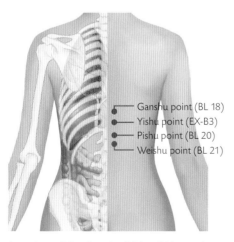

Location of the Ganshu, Yishu, Pishu and Weishu points.

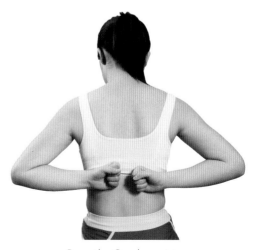

Press the Ganshu point.

5. Pressing and Kneading the Shenshu Point
Location: 1.5 cun horizontally from the second lumbar spinal process.
Method: Lie on the back or sit upright. Use the two middle fingers to forcefully press and knead the Shenshu point of both sides 30 to 50 times, keeping the thumbs by the ribs. Or, with a clenched fist, use the knuckle of the index finger to press and knead the Shenshu point 30 to 50 times. You might also try using a loose fist to knead and rub 30 to 50 times, until some warmth is felt as the best effect.
Effect: Treat waist tingling and leg pain, lumbar muscle strain, lumbar disc herniation, leg swelling, fatigue all over the body, impotence, nocturnal emission, premature ejaculation and menstrual disorder.

6. Pressing and Kneading the Yishe Point
Location: Three cun away from the spinous process of the eleventh thoracic vertebra.
Method: Sit on a chair. Use two thumbs to press and knead the Yishe points on each side respectively, with the elbow extending outward.
Effect: Cure abdominal distension, borborygmus, vomiting and diarrhea.

7. Pressing and Kneading the Sanjiaoshu Point
Location: At the point 1.5 cun away from the spinous process of the first lumbar vertebra.
Method: Sit or stand. Use two middle fingers to forcefully press and knead the Sanjiaoshu point 30 to 50 times, with thumbs grasping the ribs. You can also make a fist and use the index knuckle to press and knead 30 to 50 times. Or with hollow fists, knead and rub it 30 to 50 times, ideally until some warmth.
Effect: Adjust metabolism and overall energy, eliminate edema, thin the waist, and treat diabetes, obesity, fever, waist pain, decline of energy, acne and abnormal lumps.

8. Pressing and Kneading the Zhongwan Point
Location: In between the lower part of the sternum and the navel.
Method: Lie on the back or sit upright. First use the index or middle finger to press the point for 30 seconds. Then continue to press and knead it for two minutes, until some tingling and distension are felt.
Effect: Treat diseases of the digestive system such as constipation, abdominal distension and pain, diarrhea, borborygmus, acid regurgitation and vomiting, as well as visual dizziness, tinnitus, acne, decline of energy and neurasthenia.

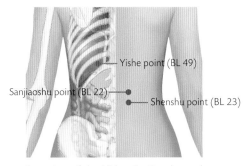
Location of the Yishe, Sanjiaoshu and Shenshu points.

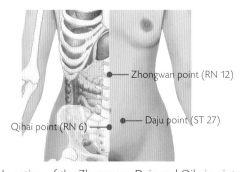
Location of the Zhongwan, Daju and Qihai points.

9. Pressing and Kneading the Qihai Point

Location: About 1.5 cun below the navel.

Method: Use the tips of the index and middle finger to press and knead the point for two minutes, until warmth is felt as the best effect.

Effect: Cure abdominal pain and distension, constipation or diarrhea, menstrual disorder, dysmenorrhea, amenorrhea, impotence, premature ejaculation and nocturnal emission.

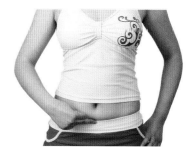

Press and knead the Qihai point.

10. Pressing and Kneading the Daju Point

Location: Two cun below the navel, two cun away from the median line.

Method: Lie on the back with knees bent. Using the four fingers of both hands, press and knead it respectively for three to five minutes.

Effect: Chiefly serve to cure distension of the lower abdomen, difficult urination, hernia, nocturnal emission, premature ejaculation, convulsion of the rectus abdominis, intestinal obstruction, cystitis and urinary retention.

11. Pressing and Kneading the Sanyinjiao Point

Location: At the rear edge of the shinbone, three cun above the ankle.

Method: Sit upright and place one shin on the opposite thigh. Use the thumb to press, rub and knead the Sanyinjiao point for about two minutes until tingling and distension are felt in the part concerned as the best effect.

Effect: Cure insomnia, palpitation, high blood pressure, menstrual disorder, dysmenorrhea, impotence and nocturnal emission.

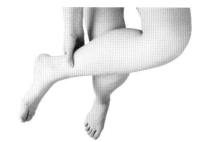

Press and knead the Sanyinjiao point.

12. Pressing the Zusanli Point

Location: About three cun below the knee on the outer side of the tibia.

Method: Sit upright. Use the tips of two thumbs to press the Zusanli point on both sides respectively for one minute with gradually increasing force.

Effect: Promote the digestion and absorption of the stomach and intestines, enhance glycogen metabolism and improve physique.

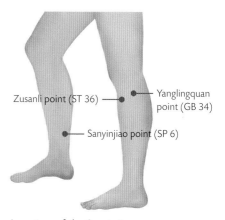

Zusanli point (ST 36)
Yanglingquan point (GB 34)
Sanyinjiao point (SP 6)

Location of the Sanyinjiao, Zusanli and Yanglingquan points.

13. Pressing and Kneading the Yanglingquan Point

Location: On the outer side of the shin in a notch at the front lower part of the fibula.

Method: Sit upright. Use the thumb tip to press the Yanglingquan point of the affected side, while putting the other four fingers at the rear of the lower leg, pressing and kneading outward for two to three minutes with slightly heavy force until some tingling and distension are obviously felt. Some patients will feel radiative numbness toward the outer side of the calf.

Effect: Treat jaundice, rib pain, bitter taste in the mouth, vomiting and acid regurgitation from liver and gallbladder problems related to gastric diseases, knee swelling and pain, lower limb paralysis and numbness, knee joint problems and febrile convulsion.

14. Pushing and Pressing the Yongquan Point

Location: In a depression in the front of the sole of the foot, about one-third of the way down from the toes.

Method: Use the small thenar (hypothenar) eminence of the left hand to forcefully and quickly push and press the Yongquan point of the right foot. Then use the small thenar eminence of the right hand to push and press the Yongquan point of

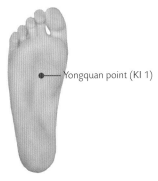

Yongquan point (KI 1)

Location of the Yongquan point.

the left foot. Keep the hand closely attached to the foot, rubbing with a higher frequency and over a longer distance, until warmth is felt in the foot sole.

Effect: Serve to speed up blood circulation of the foot sole and promotes metabolism. In addition it serves to cure foot sole pain, swelling, pale or peeling foot skin, fever, nasal discomfort, allergy, diarrhea, agitation, dizziness, insomnia, constipation and difficult urination.

Tips

- Take control over eating and drinking.
- Take medicine according to prescription. Some patients adjust the amount of glucose-reducing medicine at will, resulting in ineffective control over glucose.
- Do not discontinue use of medicine due to worry about potential side effects. Some people believe that the liver and kidneys will be harmed if medicine is taken for a long time. However generally it will be safe if the dosage is within the range stipulated by the pharmacist. Side effects only take place among a few patients and they generally disappear at once after the patient stops taking the medicine.

49 | Menstrual Disorder

Being common among women, it is featured by an unusual amount of bleeding in the cycle of menstruation or abdominal pain before and/or during menstruation, and there are often symptoms all over the body.

Irregular menstruation can be caused by blood disease, high blood pressure, liver disease, endocrine disease, abortion and ectopic pregnancy. However in most cases it is related to the disorder of endocrine functions, heavy pressure and unstable mood.

In terms of irregular menstruation, minor cases will accelerate aging, while those with severe cases will suffer from serious gynecologic diseases. Therefore women should take note of their menstrual cycle, and go to see a doctor in a timely manner when irregular menstruation occurs.

Symptoms

An abnormal cycle of menstruation and unusual amount of bleeding are attributed to several factors as follows:

• Irregular uterine bleeding: Too much blood during menstruation or a very short cycle of menstruation (less than 25 days), this often occurs with hysteromyoma (uterine fibroids) and endometriosis. Scant blood during menstruation or a very long cycle (more than 35 days).

• Dysfunctional uterine bleeding: Abnormal bleeding caused by endocrine imbalance.

• Vaginal bleeding after menopause: Bleeding six months after menopause often caused by malicious tumors and inflammation.

• Amenorrhea: No onset of menstruation at all, or the stoppage of menstruation for over three cycles after the cycle has been established.

Target Acupoints

Shoulder, back and waist: Shenshu (BL 23), Baliao (BL 31–34), Mingmen (DU 4).
Chest and abdomen: Qihai (DU 6), Guanyuan (RN 4), Zhongji (RN 3).
Legs: Xuehai (SP 10), Sanyinjiao (SP 6), Zusanli (ST 36), Yinbai (SP 1), Taichong (LV 3).

Recommended Massage

1. Pressing and Kneading the Shenshu Point
Location: 1.5 cun horizontally from the second lumbar spinal process.

Method: Lie on the back or sit upright. Use the two middle fingers to forcefully press and knead the Shenshu point of both sides 30 to 50 times, keeping the thumbs by the ribs. Or, with a clenched fist, use the knuckle of the index finger to press and knead the Shenshu point 30 to 50 times. You might also try using a loose fist to knead and rub 30 to 50 times, until some warmth is felt as the best effect.

Effect: Treat waist tingling and leg pain, lumbar muscle strain, lumbar disc herniation, leg swelling, fatigue all over the body, impotence, nocturnal emission, premature ejaculation and menstrual disorder.

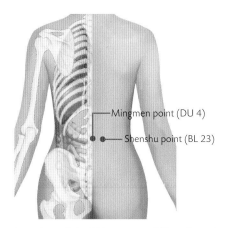
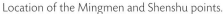

Location of the Mingmen and Shenshu points.

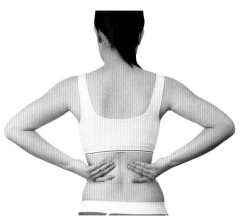

Press and knead the Shenshu point.

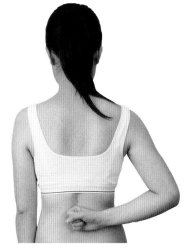

Press the Mingmen point.

2. Pressing the Mingmen Point
Location: In a cavity below the spinous process of the second cervical vertebra.

Method: Sit upright or lie on the back, with the back straightening up slightly. Use the back of the palm or the knuckles to press the point rhythmically for two minutes with a little heavier force.

Effect: Treat severe waist pain, leg paralysis, menstrual disorder, reddish leucorrhea, dysmenorrhea, amenorrhea and infertility, as well as nocturnal emission, impotence, infertility due to cold sperm, frequent urination, cold pain in the lower abdomen, and diarrhea.

3. Kneading and Rubbing the Baliao Points
Location: There are eight Baliao points in total, four on each side of the sacral spine. These are the upper, secondary, middle and lower Baliao points. They are located respectively in the first, second, third and fourth posterior sacral foramina (opening between vertebrae).

Method: Sit upright. Use the palm to knead, or rub up and down, along the sacral vertebrae for about two minutes, until some tingling and distension are felt as the best effect.

Effect: Cure pain in the lumbosacral spine, constipation, distension and pain in the lower abdomen, pelvic inflammation, difficult urination, menstrual disorder and hemorrhoids.

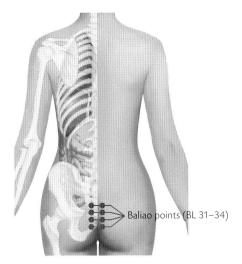
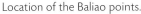

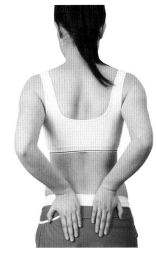

Location of the Baliao points.   Knead and rub the Baliao points.

4. Pressing and Kneading the Qihai Point

Location: About 1.5 cun below the navel.

Method: Use the tips of the index and middle finger to press and knead the point for two minutes, until warmth is felt as the best effect.

Effect: Cure abdominal pain and distension, constipation or diarrhea, menstrual disorder, dysmenorrhea, amenorrhea, impotence, premature ejaculation and nocturnal emission.

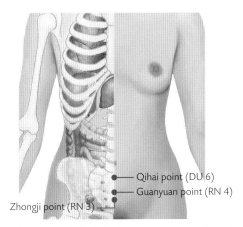

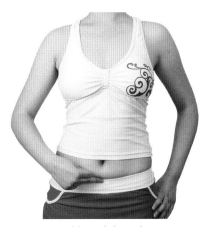

Location of the Qihai, Guanyuan and Zhongji points.   Press and knead the Qihai point.

5. Pressing and Kneading the Guanyuan Point

Location: About three cun below the navel.

Method: Sit upright or lie on the back. First use the index or middle finger to press the point for 30 seconds. Then continue to press and knead it for another two minutes, until some tingling and distension are felt as the best effect.

Effect: Cure abdominal pain and distension, menstrual disorder, dysmenorrhea, amenorrhea, nocturnal emission and impotence.

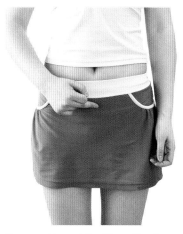

Press and knead the Zhongji point

6. Pressing and Kneading the Zhongji Point

Location: Four cun below the navel.

Method: Sit upright or lie on the back. First use the middle or index finger to press and knead the point for two minutes. Then continue to press it for another 30 seconds, until some tingling and distension are felt as the best effect.

Effect: Cure difficulty in urinating, leukorrhagia, amenorrhea, menstrual disorder, cold feeling and pain before menstruation, facial edema and lower-limb edema.

7. Pressing and Kneading the Xuehai Point

Location: In a cavity about two cun away from the inner upper corner of the patella, when the knee is bent.

Method: Sit upright. Use the pads of the thumbs to forcefully press and knead the Xuehai point of the same side for two minutes, until some tingling and distension are felt as the best effect.

Effect: Cure low blood pressure, inadequate vital energy and blood, anemia, dizziness and visual dizziness, menstrual disorder, dysmenorrhea, amenorrhea, hives, eczema, rough skin, skin itch and knee-joint pain.

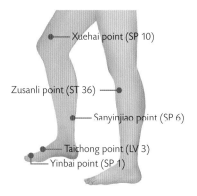

Location of the Xuehai, Zusanli, Sanyinjiao, Taichong and Yinbai points.

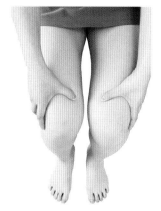

Press and knead the Xuehai point.

8. Pressing and Kneading the Sanyinjiao Point

Location: At the rear edge of the shinbone, three cun above the ankle.

Method: Sit upright and place one shin on the opposite thigh. Use the thumb to press, rub and knead the Sanyinjiao point for about two minutes until tingling and distension are felt in the part concerned as the best effect.

Effect: Cure insomnia, palpitation, high blood pressure, menstrual disorder, dysmenorrhea, impotence and nocturnal emission.

9. Pressing and Kneading the Zusanli Point

Location: About three cun below the knee on the outer side of the tibia.

Method: Sit upright. Use both thumbs to press the point on both sides, with the four fingers alongside the outer side of the lower leg, pressing and kneading outward 20 to 40 times, until some tingling and distension are felt as the best effect.

Effect: Treat diarrhea, abdominal pain and distension, lack of appetite, constipation, hiccups, vomiting, anemia, low blood pressure, menopause syndrome and waist-leg pain.

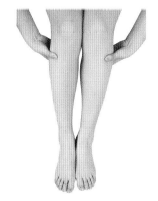

Press and knead the Zusanli point.

10. Pressing and Kneading the Taichong Point

Location: On the foot in a notch between the first and second metatarsal bones.

Method: Sit upright. Use the thumb tip to press, rub and knead the Taichong point for about two minutes and then press for another 30 seconds until tingling and distension are felt in the part concerned as the best effect.

Effect: Cure headache with distension, dizziness, migraine, menstrual disorder including dysmenorrhea and amenorrhea, and breast pain with distension.

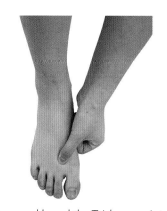

Press and knead the Taichong point.

11. Pressing the Yinbai Point

Location: Just inside the inner corner of the big toe nail.

Method: Use the thumb pad to press the point until pain is gradually felt.

Effect: Often serve to cure functional bleeding of the uterus, bleeding of the upper gastro-intestinal tract, acute enteritis, schizophrenia, neurasthenia, hypermenorrhea, hematemesis and unconsciousness.

Tips

Exposure to the cold air of the air-conditioner over a long time may lead to problems with the ovulation function, resulting in irregular menstruation, abdominal pain and distension. Therefore it is appropriate to set the indoor temperature at 26 C or so. In addition the use of air-conditioning should be controlled from one hour to three hours, or people should go out to move around once every hour.

50 | Dysmenorrhea

It refers to pain in the lower abdomen or waist during, before or after menstruation, and even pain in the lumbosacral portion. The pain lasts for one to two days or throughout the period of menstruation. Those with severe cases will suffer from it even when there is no menstruation.

Symptoms

It attacks whenever menstruation occurs. Those with severe cases will suffer from nausea, vomiting, cold sweat, cold hands and feet, and even unconsciousness, affecting work and life.

Dysmenorrhea is divided into primary and secondary cases:

Primary dysmenorrhea: It is mostly seen among young women. There is pain when menstruation starts, mostly due to mental tension or maldevelopment of the uterus.

Secondary dysmenorrhea: It is mostly caused by organic lesion of the reproductive organs, such as endometriosis, tumors and inflammation.

Target Acupoints

Shoulder, back and waist: Baliao (BL 31–34).
Chest and abdomen: Qihai (RN 6), Guanyuan (RN 4), Zhongji (RN 3).
Arms: Hegu (LI 4).
Legs: Diji (SP 8), Zusanli (ST 36), Sanyinjiao (SP 6), Dadun (LV 1), Taichong (LV 3).

Recommended Massage

1. Kneading and Rubbing the Baliao Points
Location: There are eight Baliao points in total, four on each side of the sacral spine. These are the upper, secondary, middle and lower Baliao points. They are located respectively in the first, second, third and fourth posterior sacral foramina (opening between vertebrae).

Method: Sit upright. Use the palm to knead, or rub up and down, along the sacral vertebrae for about two minutes, until some tingling and distension are felt as the best effect.

Effect: Cure pain in the lumbosacral spine, constipation, distension and pain in the lower abdomen, pelvic inflammation, difficult urination, menstrual disorder and hemorrhoids.

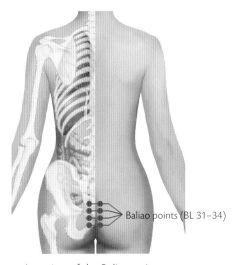

Baliao points (BL 31–34)

Location of the Baliao points.

2. Pressing and Kneading the Qihai Point

Location: About 1.5 cun below the navel.

Method: Use the tips of the index and middle finger to press and knead the point for two minutes, until warmth is felt as the best effect.

Effect: Cure abdominal pain and distension, constipation or diarrhea, menstrual disorder, dysmenorrhea, amenorrhea, impotence, premature ejaculation and nocturnal emission.

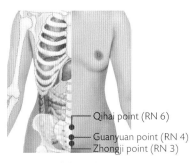

Qihai point (RN 6)
Guanyuan point (RN 4)
Zhongji point (RN 3)

Location of the Qihai, Guanyuan and Zhongji points.

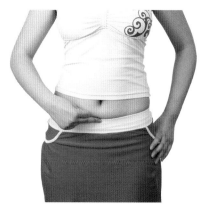

Press and knead the Qihai point.

3. Pressing and Kneading the Guanyuan Point

Location: About three cun below the navel.

Method: Sit upright or lie on the back. First use the index or middle finger to press the point for 30 seconds. Then continue to press and knead it for another two minutes, until some tingling and distension are felt as the best effect.

Effect: Cure abdominal pain and distension, menstrual disorder, dysmenorrhea, amenorrhea, nocturnal emission and impotence.

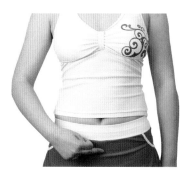

Press and knead the Guanyuan point.

4. Pressing and Kneading the Zhongji Point

Location: Four cun below the navel.

Method: Sit upright or lie on the back. Use overlapped hands to press and knead the point for two to three minutes, until some tingling and distension are felt as the best effect.

Effect: Cure difficulty in urinating, leukorrhagia, amenorrhea, menstrual disorder, cold feeling and pain before menstruation, facial edema and lower-limb edema.

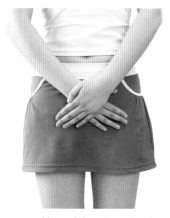

Press and knead the Zhongji point.

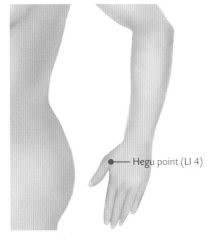

Location of the Hegu point.

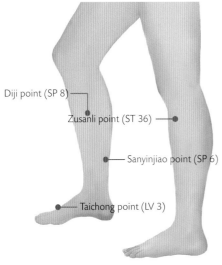

Diji point (SP 8)

Zusanli point (ST 36)

Sanyinjiao point (SP 6)

Taichong point (LV 3)

Location of the Diji, Zusanli, Sanyinjiao and Taichong point.

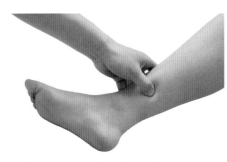

Press and knead the Sanyinjiao point.

5. Pinching and Kneading the Hegu Point

Location: In the highest point on the back of the hand between the thumb base and the base of the index finger (in the webbing between these two fingers).

Method: Sit upright or lie on the back. Use the thumb to press and knead the Hegu point while using the index finger to press its corresponding point on the palm 10 to 20 times alternately. Proceed from light to heavy force, until some tingling and distension are felt as the best effect.

Effect: Treat facioplegia, trigeminal pain, facial paralysis, deviated mouth and eyes (facial paralysis), rhinitis, headache, toothache, acne, visual fatigue, sore throat, tinnitus and hiccups.

6. Pressing and Kneading the Diji Point

Location: Three cun below the Yinlingquan point., on the line connecting the Yinlingquan point and the medial malleolus.

Method: Use two thumbs to press and knead the Diji point of the same side respectively for two minutes, proceeding from light to heavy force. Then forcefully press it for 30 seconds continually.

Effect: Treat abdominal distension and pain, diarrhea, edema, difficult urination, menstrual disorder, bacillary dysentery, dysmenorrhea, gastric convulsion, dysentery and functional bleeding of the uterus.

7. Pressing and Kneading the Sanyinjiao Point

Location: At the rear edge of the shinbone, three cun above the ankle.

Method: Sit upright and place one shin on the opposite thigh. Use the thumb to press, rub and knead the Sanyinjiao point for about two minutes until tingling and distension are felt in the part concerned as the best effect.

Effect: Cure insomnia, palpitation, high blood pressure, menstrual disorder, dysmenorrhea, impotence and nocturnal emission.

8. Pressing and Kneading the Zusanli Point

Location: About three cun below the knee on the outer side of the tibia.

Method: Sit upright. Use two thumbs to press and knead the point of the same side for two minutes, with the four fingers grasping the rear of the calf, until some tingling and distension are felt as the best effect.

Effect: Treat diarrhea, abdominal pain and distension, lack of appetite, constipation, hiccups, vomiting, anemia, low blood pressure, menopause syndrome and waist-leg pain.

9. Pressing and Kneading the Taichong Point

Location: On the foot in a notch between the first and second metatarsal bones.

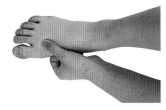

Method: Sit upright. Use the thumb tip to press and knead the Taichong point for about two minutes and then press for another 30 seconds until tingling and distension are felt in the part concerned as the best effect.

Press and knead the Taichong point.

Effect: Cure headache with distension, dizziness, migraine, menstrual disorder including dysmenorrhea and amenorrhea, and breast pain with distension.

10. Pinching and Pressing the Dadun Point

Location: At the point 0.1 cun away from the big toe nail.

Method: Use the tip of the index or middle finger to pinch and press the point for two minutes.

Effect: Treat hernia, retracted genitals, vaginal pain, menstrual disorder, profuse uterine bleeding, hematuria, difficult urination, bed-wetting, gonorrhea, epilepsy and pain in the lower abdomen.

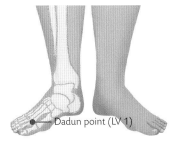

Dadun point (LV 1)

Pinch and press the Dadun point.

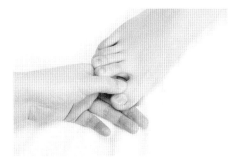

Tips
- Do more physical exercise.
- Eat nutritious food.
- Take a proactive attitude toward having chronic diseases treated.

51 Premenstrual Tension

Women suffering from it tend to experience a number of uncomfortable symptoms one to two weeks before menstruation,mostly marked by anxiety. It may be associated with protracted irritation, endocrine disorder or imbalance of hormone levels. It is mostly seen among women aged from 30 to 40.

Symptoms

Typical premenstrual tension takes place one week before menstruation, with a series of symptoms of different degrees such as mental tension, depression, agitation, insomnia and diarrhea, as well as dread of the onset of menstruation. The symptoms gradually become worse and will be the worst two to three days before menstruation. Then they will disappear suddenly after menstruation begins. However in some women symptoms continue for quite a long time, and will not disappear completely three to four days after menstruation starts.

Target Acupoints

Head and neck: Taitang (EX-HN 5).
Shoulder, back and waist: Shenshu (BL 23), Xinshu (BL 15), Ganshu (BL 18).
Chest and abdomen: Danzhong (RN 17), Guanyuan (RN 4).
Arms: Neiguan (PC 6), Laogong (PC 8).
Legs: Sanyinjiao (SP 6), Taichong (LV 3).

Recommended Massage

1. Pressing and Kneading the Shenshu Point
Location: 1.5 cun horizontally from the second lumbar spinal process.
   Method: Lie on the back or sit upright. Use the two middle fingers to forcefully press and knead the Shenshu point of both sides 30 to 50 times, keeping the thumbs by the ribs. Or, with a clenched fist, use the knuckle of the index finger to press and

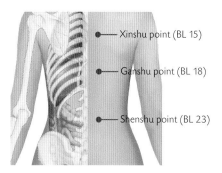

Location of the Xinshu, Ganshu and Shenshu points.

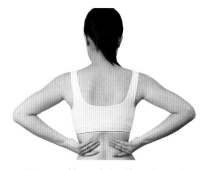

Press and knead the Shenshu point.

knead the Shenshu point 30 to 50 times. You might also try using a loose fist to knead and rub 30 to 50 times, until some warmth is felt as the best effect.

Effect: Treat waist tingling and leg pain, lumbar muscle strain, lumbar disc herniation, leg swelling, fatigue all over the body, impotence, nocturnal emission, premature ejaculation and menstrual disorder.

2. Pressing the Ganshu Point

Location: 1.5 cun away from the ninth thoracic spinal process on the inner side of the scapula.

Method: Sit upright. Use the knuckles of the four fingers to knead the Ganshu point for about two minutes until tingling and distension are felt.

Effect: Treat distension and pain of both sides of the chest, breast pain with swelling, waist-back pain, agitation, irritability, indigestion and aversion to food, neurasthenia, hepatitis, jaundice (icterus), nausea, vomiting, lack of appetite and dizziness.

3. Pressing and Kneading the Xinshu Point

Location: Under the fifth thoracic vertebra on the inner side of the scapula, 1.5 cun horizontally away.

Method: Sit on a chair. Use the middle finger to press and knead the Xinshu point for about two minutes, until tingling and distension are felt.

Effect: Treat agitation, palpitation, difficulty breathing, heart pain, cough, hematemesis, chest-back pain, insomnia, forgetfulness, night sweating, wet dream and epilepsy.

4. Pressing and Kneading the Guanyuan Point

Location: About three cun below the navel.

Method: Sit upright or lie on the back. First use the index or middle finger to press the point for two minutes. Then continue to press and knead it for another 30 seconds, until some tingling and distension are felt as the best effect.

Effect: Cure abnormal leucorrhoea, abdominal pain before menstruation, abdominal distension, diarrhea, amenorrhea, infertility, bed-wetting, frequent urination, urine retention, dizziness and headache.

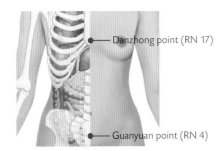
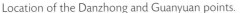
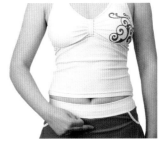

Location of the Danzhong and Guanyuan points.   Press and knead the Guanyuan point.

5. Palm Kneading the Danzhong Point

Location: Directly in the middle of the chest between the nipples.

Method: Use the thenar eminence of the left hand or the palm heel against the

Danzhong point, kneading it 30 to 40 times. Then use the right hand to knead 30 to 40 times, until distension and numbness radiate to the chest as the best effect.

Effect: Cure difficulty in breathing, anxiety, palpitation, cough, chest pain, hyperplasia of the mammary glands, breast pain, lactation deficiency and obesity.

6. Pressing and Kneading the Taiyang Point

Location: In the depression about one cun behind the space between the outer tip of the brow and outer eye corner.

Method: Sit upright or lie on the back. Use the pad of the index finger to press the Taiyang points on both sides of the head, rubbing and kneading for two minutes until you feel tingling and expansion in the acupoints. If rubbing and kneading of a larger area is required, or you need more force, use the thenar eminences.

Effect: Cure cold, headache, fever, dizziness, and red and swollen eyes with pain.

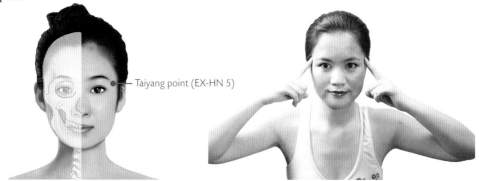

Press and knead the Taiyang point.

7. Pushing and Kneading the Laogong Point

Location: With the fingers curled in toward the palm, the point reached by the tip of the middle finger into the palm.

Method: Use the thumb to push and knead the point in all directions for two minutes, using two hands alternately, until some tingling and distension are felt as the best effect.

Effect: Promote blood circulation in the hands, adjust metabolism, reduce palm fat, reinforce the flexibility and elasticity of the joints and muscles of the hands, and cure apoplexy, unconsciousness, heat-stroke, heart pain, epilepsy, oral ulcer and bad breath.

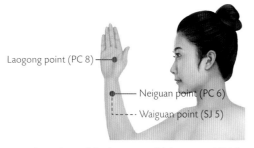

Location of the Laogong, Neiguan and Waiguan points.

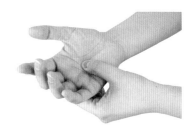

Push and knead the Laogong point.

8. Pressing and Kneading the Neiguan and Waiguan Points

Location: Between the two tendons about two cun above the wrist joint bend.

Method: Bend the forearm halfway. Use the thumb tip of one hand to press the Neiguan point while using the index or middle finger to press the Waiguan point, pressing inward 20 to 30 times.

Effect: Cure vomiting, hiccups, chest distress, chest pain, insomnia, agitation, palpitation, gastritis, gastric ulcer, heat-stroke and migraine.

9. Pressing and Kneading the Sanyinjiao Point

Location: At the rear edge of the shinbone, three cun above the ankle.

Method: Sit upright and place one shin on the opposite thigh. Use the thumb to press, rub and knead the Sanyinjiao point for about two minutes until tingling and distension are felt in the part concerned as the best effect.

Effect: Cure insomnia, palpitation, high blood pressure, menstrual disorder, dysmenorrhea, impotence and nocturnal emission.

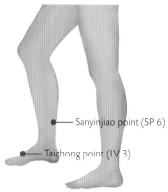

Sanyinjiao point (SP 6)

Taichong point (IV 3)

Location of the Sanyinjiao and Taichong points.

10. Pressing and Kneading the Taichong Point

Location: On the foot in a notch between the first and second metatarsal bones.

Method: Sit upright. Use the thumb tip to press, rub and knead the Taichong point for about two minutes and then press for another 30 seconds until tingling and distension are felt in the part concerned as the best effect.

Effect: Cure headache with distension, dizziness, migraine, menstrual disorder including dysmenorrhea and amenorrhea, and breast pain with distension.

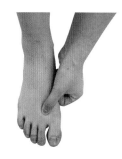

Press and knead the Taichong point.

Tips
- Do more physical exercise, particularly regular aerobic exercise of moderate strength, such as jogging and swimming.
- Adjust the amount of exercise according to physiological condition. For instance it is appropriate for office workers to take a brisk walk of two to three kilometers, four to five times each week, and then gradually increase the amount of exercise.
- Persistence is most important.

52 | Amenorrhea

It refers to the condition when women fail to start menstruation after 18 years old, or fail to have it for a period of over three months after onset of menstruation. Primary amenorrhea is found in women without menstruation by the age of 18, while secondary amenorrhea is found in women without menstruation after 18.

Amenorrhea may be caused by abnormal endocrine function or dysfunction of the reproductive organs. In the latter case it cannot be treated by massage, and therefore requires timely medical treatment.

Symptoms

In addition to absence of menstruation, amenorrhea is accompanied by dizziness, tinnitus, tingling in the waist and weakness in the legs.

Target Acupoints

Shoulder, back and waist: Ganshu (BL 18), Weishu (BL 21), Pishu (BL 20), Shenshu (BL 23).
Chest and abdomen: Qihai (RN 6), Guilai (ST 29), Guanyuan (RN 4), Zigong (EX-CA 1).
Legs: Xuehai (SP 10), Sanyinjiao (SP 6), Gongsun (SP 4), Rangu (KI 2).

Recommended Massage

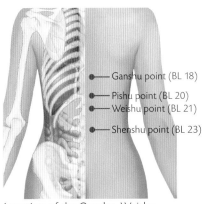

Ganshu point (BL 18)
Pishu point (BL 20)
Weishu point (BL 21)
Shenshu point (BL 23)

Location of the Ganshu, Weishu, Pishu and Shenshu points.

1. Pressing the Ganshu Point
Location: 1.5 cun away from the ninth thoracic spinal process on the inner side of the scapula.

Method: Sit upright. Use the knuckles of the four fingers to knead the Ganshu point for about two minutes until tingling and distension are felt.

Effect: Treat distension and pain of both sides of the chest, breast pain with swelling, waist-back pain, agitation, irritability, indigestion and aversion to food, neurasthenia, hepatitis, jaundice (icterus), nausea, vomiting, lack of appetite and dizziness.

2. Pressing and Kneading the Weishu Point
Location: About 1.5 cun below the spinous process of the twelfth thoracic vertebra.

Method: Sit or stand. Use the middle fingers to press and knead the Weishu point of both sides (with the thumb against the ribs) forcefully for two minutes. Alternately make a fist and use the protruding index knuckle to press and knead it for two minutes. Or with a loose fist, press and rub the point for two minutes. In all cases some tingling and distension are felt as the best effect.

Effect: Treat all kinds of diseases and symptoms of the digestive system, such as acute gastritis, chronic gastritis, gastroptosis, stomach atony, abdominal distension, abdominal pain, lack of appetite, nausea and vomiting.

3. Pressing and Kneading the Pishu Point

Location: At the point 1.5 cun away horizontally from the eleventh thoracic vertebra.

Method: Sit or stand. Use both middle fingers to press the Pishu point, with the thumb against the ribs, forcefully pressing and kneading for two minutes. Or with a clenched fist, use the index knuckle to press and knead the Pishu point for two minutes. Alternatively you may use a hollow fist to knead and rub it for two minutes, until some tingling and distension are felt.

Effect: Cure nausea, vomiting, abdominal distension, diarrhea, hemafecia (bloody stool) and jaundice.

4. Pressing and Kneading the Shenshu Point

Location: 1.5 cun horizontally from the second lumbar spinal process.

Method: Lie on the back or sit upright. Use the two middle fingers to forcefully press and knead the Shenshu point of both sides 30 to 50 times, keeping the thumbs by the ribs. Or, with a clenched fist, use the knuckle of the index finger to press and knead the Shenshu point 30 to 50 times. You might also try using a loose fist to knead and rub 30 to 50 times, until some warmth is felt as the best effect.

Effect: Treat waist tingling and leg pain, lumbar muscle strain, lumbar disc herniation, leg swelling, fatigue all over the body, impotence, nocturnal emission, premature ejaculation and menstrual disorder.

5. Pressing and Kneading the Qihai Point

Location: About 1.5 cun below the navel.

Method: Sit upright or lie on the back. Use the middle finger to press and knead the point for two to three minutes, until warmth is felt as the best effect.

Effect: Cure abdominal pain and distension, constipation or diarrhea, menstrual disorder, dysmenorrhea and amenorrhea.

6. Pressing and Kneading the Guilai Point

Location: Four cun below the navel and two cun away from the frontal middle line.

Method: Sit upright or lie on the back. Use two middle fingers to press and knead the Guilai points of both sides for two minutes. Then continue to press for another 30 seconds, until some tingling and distension are felt, ideally radiating to the entire abdomen.

Effect: Treat infertility, amenorrhea, menstrual disorder, dysmenorrhea, uterus prolapse, appendicitis and pelvic inflammation.

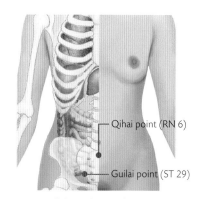

Location of the Qihai and Guilai points.

7. Pressing and Kneading the Guanyuan Point

Location: About three cun below the navel.

Method: Use two palms to press and knead the point for three minutes, until warmth is felt in the abdomen.

Effect: Cure abdominal pain and distension, menstrual disorder, dysmenorrhea, amenorrhea, nocturnal emission and impotence.

8. Pressing and Kneading the Zigong Point

Location: Four cun below the navel and three cun away from the frontal middle line.

Method: Sit upright or lie on the back. First use the index or middle finger to press the point for two minutes. Then continue to press and knead it for another 30 seconds, until some tingling and distension are felt as the best effect.

Effect: Treat dysmenorrhea, menstrual disorder, profuse uterine bleeding, infertility and uterus prolapse.

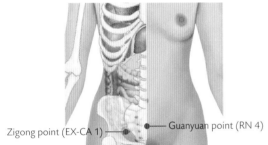

Zigong point (EX-CA 1) —   — Guanyuan point (RN 4)

Location of the Guanyuan and Zigong points.

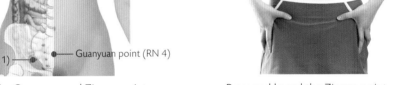

Press and knead the Zigong point.

9. Pressing and Kneading the Xuehai Point

Location: In a cavity about two cun away from the inner upper corner of the patella, when the knee is bent.

Method: Sit upright. Use the pads of the thumbs to forcefully press and knead the Xuehai point of the same side for two minutes, until some tingling and distension are felt as the best effect.

Effect: Cure low blood pressure, inadequate vital energy and blood, anemia, dizziness and visual dizziness, menstrual disorder, dysmenorrhea, amenorrhea, hives, eczema, rough skin, skin itch and knee-joint pain.

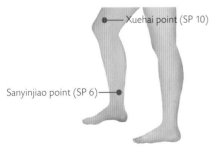

— Xuehai point (SP 10)

Sanyinjiao point (SP 6) —

Location of the Xuehai and Sanyinjiao points.

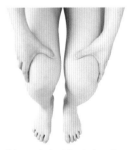

Press and knead the Xuehai point.

10. Pressing and Kneading the Sanyinjiao Point

Location: At the rear edge of the shinbone, three cun above the ankle.

Method: Sit upright and place one shin on the opposite thigh. Use the thumb to press, rub and knead the Sanyinjiao point for about two minutes until tingling and distension are felt in the part concerned as the best effect.

Effect: Cure insomnia, palpitation, high blood pressure, menstrual disorder and dysmenorrhea.

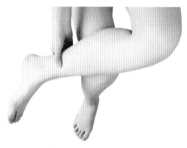

Press and knead the Sanyinjiao point.

11. Pressing and Kneading the Gongsun Point

Location: At the point of the frontal lower part at the base of the first metatarsal bone.

Method: Sit upright. Use the thumb tip to press and knead the point for two minutes and then continue to press it for another 30 seconds, until tingling and distension are felt as the best effect.

Effect: Treat acute gastritis, gastric convulsion, intestinal convulsion, acute enteritis, nervous vomiting, diaphragm spasm, the aftereffect of myocarditis, pleurisy, peritonitis, head-face edema, epilepsy, ascites due to cirrhosis, malaria, leg paralysis and inflammation at the inguinal lymph nodes.

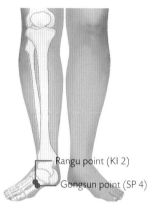

Rangu point (KI 2)

Gongsun point (SP 4)

Location of the Rangu and Gaongsun points.

12. Pressing the Rangu Point

Location: On the inner side of the foot directly above the arch, up halfway to the top of the foot.

Method: Sit upright. Use the thumb tip to press the point, until some tingling and distension are felt.

Effect: Often serves to cure acute and chronic gastritis, ulcer of the digestive system, acute and chronic enteritis, nervous vomiting, indigestion and schizophrenia. In coordination with the Zhongwan point and Zusanli point, it can cure gastric distension and pain. In coordination with the Fenglong point and Danzhong point, it can cure vomiting and visual dizziness.

Tips
- Keep a light-hearted mood, avoid excessive mental tension and reduce irritation.
- Adjust diet and pay attention to the intake of protein and other nutritious food.
- Avoid excessive food reduction or weight loss.

53 | Chronic Pelvic Inflammation

It refers to chronic inflammation of the inner reproductive organs and the surrounding connective tissues and pelvic peritoneum. It usually occurs as a result of childbirth, abortion or abdominal operation. Due to improper treatment of acute infection, some women suffer from pelvic inflammation that can never be cured.

Symptoms

It is mainly marked by continuous and distended pain in the lower abdomen, and tingling and pain in the lower waist generally accompanied by frequent, urgent or difficult urination. Those with severe cases suffer from high fever, chills, headache and lack of appetite, along with leucorrhea (vaginal discharge) of a large amount and bad odor.

Target Acupoints

Shoulder, back and waist: Ganshu (BL 18), Shenshu (BL 23), Baliao (BL 31–34).
Chest and abdomen: Guanyuan (RN 4), Zigong (EX-CA 1), Zhongji (RN 3), Guilai (ST 29).
Arms: Xuehai (SP 10), Sanyinjiao (SP 6), Zusanli (ST 36).

Recommended Massage

1. Pressing the Ganshu Point
Location: 1.5 cun away from the ninth thoracic spinal process on the inner side of the scapula.

 Method: Sit upright. Use the knuckles of the four fingers to knead the Ganshu point for about two minutes until tingling and distension are felt.

 Effect: Treat distension and pain of both sides of the chest, breast pain with swelling, waist-back pain, agitation, irritability, indigestion and aversion to food, neurasthenia, hepatitis, jaundice (icterus), nausea, vomiting, lack of appetite and dizziness.

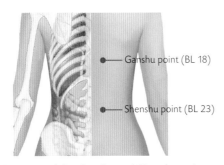

Location of the Ganshu and Shenshu points.

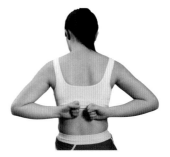

Press the Ganshu point.

2. Pressing and Kneading the Shenshu Point

Location: 1.5 cun horizontally from the second lumbar spinal process.

Method: Lie on the back or sit upright. Use the two middle fingers to forcefully press and knead the Shenshu point of both sides 30 to 50 times, keeping the thumbs by the ribs. Or, with a clenched fist, use the knuckle of the index finger to press and knead the Shenshu point 30 to 50 times. You might also try using a loose fist to knead and rub 30 to 50 times, until some warmth is felt as the best effect.

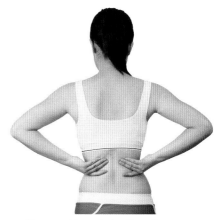

Press and knead the Shenshu point.

Effect: Treat waist tingling and leg pain, lumbar muscle strain, lumbar disc herniation, leg swelling, fatigue all over the body, impotence, nocturnal emission, premature ejaculation and menstrual disorder.

3. Kneading and Rubbing the Baliao Points

Location: There are eight Baliao points in total, four on each side of the sacral spine. These are the upper, secondary, middle and lower Baliao points. They are located respectively in the first, second, third and fourth posterior sacral foramina (opening between vertebrae).

Method: Sit upright. Use the palm to knead, or rub up and down, along the sacral vertebrae for about two minutes, until some tingling and distension are felt as the best effect.

Effect: Cure pain in the lumbosacral spine, constipation, distension and pain in the lower abdomen, pelvic inflammation, difficult urination, menstrual disorder and hemorrhoids.

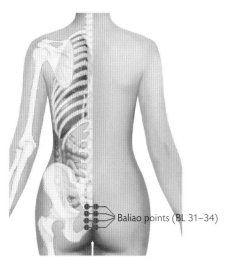
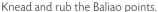

Baliao points (BL 31–34)

Knead and rub the Baliao points.

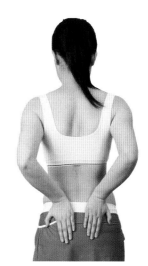

4. Pressing and Kneading the Guanyuan Point
Location: About three cun below the navel.
　　Method: Use two palms to press and knead the point for three minutes, until warmth is felt in the abdomen.
　　Effect: Cure abdominal pain and distension, menstrual disorder, dysmenorrhea, amenorrhea, nocturnal emission and impotence.

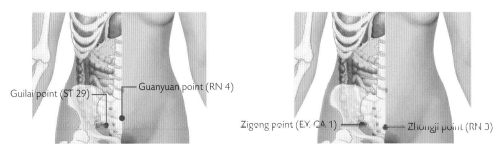

Location of the Guilai, Zigong, Guanyuan and Zhongji Points.

5. Pressing and Kneading the Guilai Point
Location: Four cun below the navel and two cun away from the frontal middle line.
　　Method: Sit upright or lie on the back. Use two middle fingers to press and knead the Guilai points of both sides for two minutes. Then continue to press for another 30 seconds, until some tingling and distension are felt, ideally radiating to the entire abdomen.
　　Effect: Treat infertility, amenorrhea, menstrual disorder, dysmenorrhea, uterus prolapse, appendicitis and pelvic inflammation.

6. Pressing and Kneading the Zhongji Point
Location: Four cun below the navel.
　　Method: Sit upright or lie on the back. First use the middle or index finger to press and knead the point for two minutes. Then continue to press it for another 30 seconds, until some tingling and distension are felt as the best effect.
　　Effect: Cure difficulty in urinating, leukorrhagia, amenorrhea, menstrual disorder, cold feeling and pain before menstruation, facial edema and lower-limb edema.

7. Pressing and Kneading the Zigong Point
Location: Four cun below the navel and three cun away from the frontal middle line.
　　Method: Sit upright or lie on the back. Use two thumbs to press and knead the Zigong points of both sides for two minutes. Then continue to press for another 30 seconds, until some tingling and distension are felt, ideally radiating to the entire abdomen.
　　Effect: Treat dysmenorrhea, menstrual disorder, profuse uterine bleeding, infertility and uterus prolapse.

8. Pressing and Kneading the Xuehai Point
Location: In a cavity about two cun away from the inner upper corner of the patella, when the knee is bent.

Method: Sit upright. Use the pads of the thumbs to forcefully press and knead the Xuehai point of the same side for two minutes, until some tingling and distension are felt as the best effect.

Effect: Cure low blood pressure, inadequate vital energy and blood, anemia, dizziness and visual dizziness, menstrual disorder, dysmenorrhea, amenorrhea, hives, eczema, rough skin, skin itch and knee-joint pain.

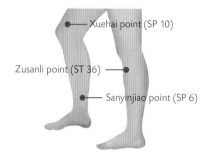

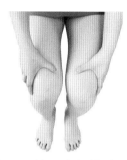

Location of the Xuehai, Zusanli and Sanyinjiao points.   Press and knead the Xuehai point.

9. Pressing and Kneading the Sanyinjiao Point

Location: At the rear edge of the shinbone, three cun above the ankle.

Method: Sit upright and place one shin on the opposite thigh. Use the thumb to press, rub and knead the Sanyinjiao point for about two minutes until tingling and distension are felt in the part concerned as the best effect.

Effect: Cure insomnia, palpitation, high blood pressure, menstrual disorder, dysmenorrhea, impotence and nocturnal emission.

10. Pressing and Kneading the Zusanli Point

Location: About three cun below the knee on the outer side of the tibia.

Method: Sit upright. Use both thumbs to press the point on both sides, with the four fingers alongside the outer side of the lower leg, pressing and kneading outward 20 to 40 times, until some tingling and distension are felt as the best effect.

Effect: Treat diarrhea, abdominal pain and distension, lack of appetite, constipation, hiccups, vomiting, anemia, low blood pressure, menopause syndrome and waist-leg pain.

Tips

Patients with chronic pelvic inflammation must receive timely and thorough treatment. To achieve a cure the patient must follow the doctor's advice regarding the right medicine, and taking medicine without guidance is prohibited. At present the combination of physical treatment with medicine is utilized with most patients.

Patients who fail to receive timely treatment often suffer from fallopian tube issues leading to infertility.

54 | Abnormal Leucorrhea

Under normal conditions, there is a little odor-free leucorrhea inside and outside the vagina. The quality and quantity are associated with the woman's physiological state. If there is too much leucorrhea or it is abnormal, it is called pathologic leucorrhea.

There are many causes for abnormal leucorrhea such as various kinds of gynecologic inflammation.

Symptoms

In clinical practice, there are several kinds of pathologic leucorrhea:

Colorless, transparent and sticky leucorrhea: It looks like egg white or is slightly turbid. Otherwise there will be no other symptoms. It often takes place in cases of chronic cervicitis, cervical canal inflammation and after estrogenic hormone is used.

Spongy leucorrhea: It is unique to colpitis mycotica. The vagina is often covered with a layer of white membrane inside and outside, with red and swollen mucosa exposed after rubbing. It is often accompanied by vulva itching and burning pain.

Yellow leucorrhea: It is mostly caused by viral infection.

Watery leucorrhea: There will be an increase of watery leucorrhea if the patient suffers from early-stage cancer, cervical cancer or tubal cancer.

Bloody leucorrhea: This is likely to be related to cancer, such as cervical cancer, cancer of the endometrium and vaginal tumor.

Yellowish and sticky leucorrhea: It is seen in cervix erosion and chronic cervicitis, caused by slight infection.

White sticky leucorrhea: Similar to normal leucorrhea but with increased amount. It takes place after estrogen is used or when there is pelvic congestion caused by the increase of secretion of the cervical glands and vaginal mucosa.

Target Acupoints

Shoulder, back and waist: Shenshu (BL 23), Mingmen (DU 4), Baliao (BL 31–34).
Chest and abdomen: Daimai (GB 26), Guanyuan (RN 4), Zigong (EX-CA 1), Zhongji (RN 3).
Legs: Yinlingquan (SP 9), Sanyinjiao (SP 6), Zusanli (ST 36), Fenglong (ST 40).

Recommended Massage
1. Pressing and Kneading the Shenshu Point
Location: 1.5 cun horizontally from the second lumbar spinal process.

Method: Lie on the back or sit upright. Use the two middle fingers to forcefully press and knead the Shenshu point of both sides 30 to 50 times, keeping the thumbs by the ribs. Or, with a clenched fist, use the knuckle of the index finger to press and knead the Shenshu point 30 to 50 times. You might also try using a loose fist to knead and rub 30 to 50 times, until some warmth is felt as the best effect.

Effect: Treat waist tingling and leg pain, lumbar muscle strain, lumbar disc herniation, leg swelling, fatigue all over the body, impotence, nocturnal emission, premature ejaculation and menstrual disorder.

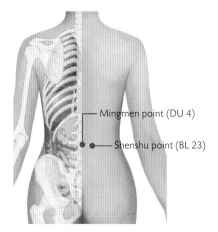
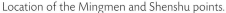

Location of the Mingmen and Shenshu points.

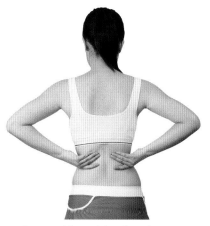

Press and knead the Shenshu point.

2. Pressing the Mingmen Point
Location: In a cavity below the spinous process of the second cervical vertebra.

Method: Sit upright or lie on the back, with the back straightening up slightly. Use the back of the palm or the knuckles to press the point rhythmically for two minutes with a little heavier force.

Effect: Treat severe waist pain, leg paralysis, menstrual disorder, reddish leucorrhea, dysmenorrhea, amenorrhea and infertility, as well as cold pain in the lower abdomen, and diarrhea.

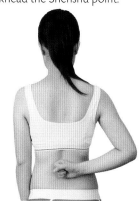

Press the Mingmen point.

3. Kneading and Rubbing the Baliao Points
Location: There are eight Baliao points in total, four on each side of the sacral spine. These are the upper, secondary, middle and lower Baliao points. They are located respectively in the first, second, third and fourth posterior sacral foramina (opening between vertebrae).

Method: Sit upright. Use the palm to knead, or rub up and down, along the sacral vertebrae for about two minutes, until some tingling and distension are felt as the best effect.

Effect: Cure pain in the lumbosacral spine, constipation, distension and pain in the lower abdomen, pelvic inflammation, difficult urination, menstrual disorder and hemorrhoids.

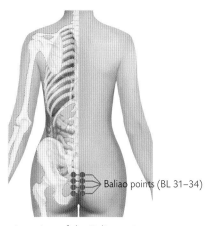

Location of the Baliao points.

4. Pressing and Kneading the Guanyuan Point

Location: About three cun below the navel.

Method: Sit upright or lie on the back. First use the index or middle finger to press the point for two minutes. Then continue to press it for another 30 seconds, until some tingling and distension are felt as the best effect.

Effect: Cure abnormal leucorrhoea, abdominal pain before menstruation, abdominal distension, diarrhea, amenorrhea, infertility, bed-wetting, frequent urination, urine retention, dizziness and headache.

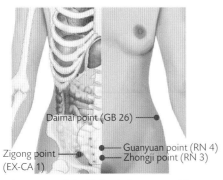

Location of the Daimai, Guanyuan, Zigong and Zhongji points.

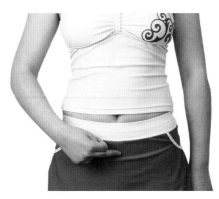

Press and knead the Guanyuan point.

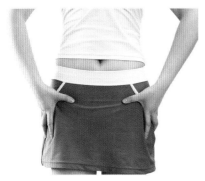

Press and knead the Zigong point.

5. Pressing and Kneading the Zigong Point

Location: Four cun below the navel and three cun away from the frontal middle line.

Method: Sit upright or lie on the back. Use two thumbs to press and knead the Zigong points of both sides for two minutes. Then continue to press for another 30 seconds, until some tingling and distension are felt, ideally radiating to the entire abdomen.

Effect: Treat dysmenorrhea, menstrual disorder, profuse uterine bleeding, infertility and uterus prolapse.

6. Pressing and Kneading the Daimai Point

Location: At the crossing of a vertical line from the frontal end of the eleventh rib with a horizontal line through the navel.

Method: Stand or lie on the back. Use two middle fingers to press and knead the Daimai point of both sides for two minutes, until some tingling and distension are felt.

Effect: Cure menstrual disorder, excess or odorous leucorrhoea, hernia, waist-back weakness and chest pain.

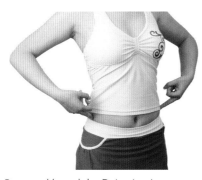

Press and knead the Daimai point.

7. Pressing and Kneading the Zhongji Point

Location: Four cun below the navel.

Method: Sit upright or lie on the back. First use the middle finger of the right hand to press and knead the point for two minutes, and then continue to press it for another 30 seconds, until some tingling and distension are felt.

Effect: Cure difficulty in urinating, leukorrhagia, amenorrhea, menstrual disorder, cold feeling and pain before menstruation, facial edema and lower-limb edema.

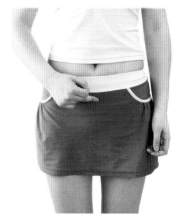

Press and knead the Zhongji point.

8. Pressing and Kneading the Yinlingquan Point

Location: In the depression on the inner edge of the shinbone below the knee.

Method: Sit upright. Use the thumb tip to press and knead the point for two minutes, and then continue to press it for another 30 seconds, until tingling and distension are felt as the best effect.

Effect: Cure knee joint swelling and pain, abdominal distension, diarrhea, obesity, facial edema or edema all over the body, yellowish skin, difficult urination or incontinence, menstrual disorder and increase of abnormal leucorrhea.

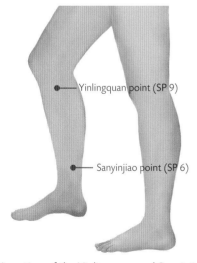

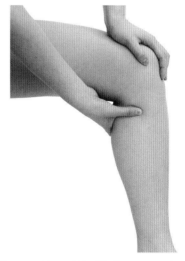

Yinlingquan point (SP 9)

Sanyinjiao point (SP 6)

Location of the Yinlingquan and Sanyinjiao points.   Press and knead the Yinlingquan point.

9. Pressing and Kneading the Sanyinjiao Point

Location: At the rear edge of the shinbone, three cun above the ankle.

Method: Sit upright and place one shin on the opposite thigh. Use the thumb to press, rub and knead the Sanyinjiao point for about two minutes until tingling and distension are felt in the part concerned as the best effect.

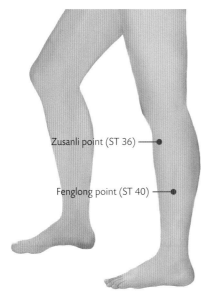

Location of the Zusanli and Fenglong points.

Effect: Cure insomnia, palpitation, high blood pressure, menstrual disorder, dysmenorrhea, impotence and noctyrnal emission.

10. Pressing and Kneading the Fenglong Point

Location: Eight cun above the ankle tip.

Method: Sit upright. Use the thumb pad to press and knead the Fenglong points on both sides for two minutes, until tingling and distension are felt as the best effect.

Effect: Chiefly serve to treat mental disorders such as hysteria, insomnia and headache, as well as diseases of the circulatory system, such as high blood pressure, cerebral hemorrhage and the aftereffect of cerebrovascular diseases. It is beneficial for diseases of the respiratory system, such as acute and chronic bronchitis, asthma and pleurisy, as well as diseases of the digestive system, such as hepatitis, appendicitis, and constipation. In addition it can cure urine retention, addiction to smoking, obesity, leg-knee tingling and pain, and shoulder periarthritis.

11. Pressing and Kneading the Zusanli Point

Location: About three cun below the knee on the outer side of the tibia.

Method: Sit upright. Use both thumbs to press the point on both sides, with the four fingers alongside the outer side of the lower leg, pressing and kneading outward 20 to 40 times, until some tingling and distension are felt as the best effect.

Effect: Treat diarrhea, abdominal pain and distension, lack of appetite, constipation, hiccups, vomiting, anemia, low blood pressure, menopause syndrome and waist-leg pain.

Tips

When leucorrhea is found, attention should first be paid to whether it is due to a physiological change. Treatment is needed as soon as possible if the amount or state is outside the normal range. This is particularly the case when women are in the climacteric period or menopause, when tumors are most likely, so as to uncover disease in time for appropriate treatment. It is absolutely prohibited for patients to self-prescribe, so as not to delay correct medical diagnosis and treatment.

55 Vulva Itching

It is caused by various pathological changes on the vulva. However it can also happen to women with completely normal vulva. Patients will feel anxious when the itching becomes worse, even to the extent of affecting life and work. When it attacks patients should first see a doctor to find out the cause and receive treatment accordingly.

Symptoms

It takes place mostly on the clitoris and labium minus, and may also affect the labium majus pudendi, perineum and anus, which are apt to be subject to abrasion. Such itching is uncontrollable and may be continuous.

It becomes worse during menstruation, at night or after eating irritating food. Such itching is generally paroxysmal but may affect sleep and study seriously. Usually it becomes worse at night.

Vulva itching without any reason mostly happens to women at childbearing age or after menopause. It can affect the entire vagina, or a certain part of it, or one side of the vulva. Though the itching is quite serious and even unbearable, the affected part and mucosa look normal, or there are only marks due to excessive scratching.

Target Acupoints

Shoulder, back and waist: Pishu (BL 20), Shenshu (BL 23).
Chest and abdomen: Huiyin (RN 1), Qugu (RN 2), Guilai (ST 29), Shuidao (ST 28), Zhongji (RN 3).
Legs: Baichongwo (EX-LE 3), Zusanli (ST 36), Sanyinjiao (SP 6), Xuehai (SP 10).

Recommended Massage

1. Pressing and Kneading the Pishu Point
Location: At the point 1.5 cun away horizontally from the eleventh thoracic vertebra.

Method: Sit or stand. Use both middle fingers to press the Pishu point, with the thumb against the ribs, forcefully pressing and kneading for two minutes. Or with a clenched fist, use the index knuckle to press and knead the Pishu point for two minutes. Alternatively you may use a hollow fist to knead and rub it for two minutes, until some tingling and distension are felt.

Effect: Cure nausea, vomiting, abdominal distension, diarrhea, hemafecia (bloody stool) and jaundice.

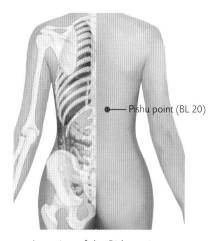

Pishu point (BL 20)

Location of the Pishu point.

2. Pressing and Kneading the Shenshu Point

Location: 1.5 cun horizontally from the second lumbar spinal process.

Method: Lie on the back or sit upright. Use the two middle fingers to forcefully press and knead the Shenshu point of both sides 30 to 50 times, keeping the thumbs by the ribs. Or, with a clenched fist, use the knuckle of the index finger to press and knead the Shenshu point 30 to 50 times. You might also try using a loose fist to knead and rub 30 to 50 times, until some warmth is felt as the best effect.

Effect: Treat waist tingling and leg pain, lumbar muscle strain, lumbar disc herniation, leg swelling, fatigue all over the body, impotence, nocturnal emission, premature ejaculation and menstrual disorder.

3. Pressing and Kneading the Huiyin Point

Location: In the middle between the anus and external genitalia.

Method: Lie on the back. Use the index or middle finger to press and knead the point for three to five minutes, until some tingling and distension are felt.

Effect: Adjust urine and excrement as well as cure hemorrhoids, vaginal pain, genital itch, genital sweating and dampness, proctoptosis, uterus prolapse and menstrual disorder.

4. Pressing and Kneading the Zhongji Point

Location: Four cun below the navel.

Method: Sit upright or lie on the back. First use the middle finger of the right hand to press and knead the point for two minutes, and then continue to press it for another 30 seconds, until some tingling and distension are felt.

Effect: Cure difficulty in urinating, leukorrhagia, amenorrhea, menstrual disorder, cold feeling and pain before menstruation, facial edema and lower-limb edema.

5. Pressing and Kneading the Qugu Point

Location: Right on the frontal line, down from the navel at the upper line of the pubic bone.

Method: Sit upright or lie on the back. Put the right palm heel on the Qugu point while placing the left palm heel on the back of the right hand. Press and knead for two minutes, until some tingling and distension are felt.

Effect: Treat menstrual disorder, uterine prolapse, urethritis, urine retention, endometritis, cervix erosion, chronic pelvic inflammation, uterine inertia, dysmenorrhea, amenorrhea and leukorrhagia.

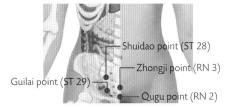

Location of the Guilai, Shuidao, Zhongji and Qugu points.

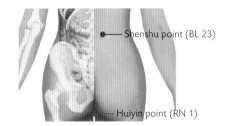

Location of the Shenshu and Huiyin points.

6. Pressing and Kneading the Guilai Point

Location: Four cun below the navel and two cun away from the frontal middle line.

Method: Sit upright or lie on the back. First use two middle fingers to press and knead the Guilai point respectively for two minutes. Then continue for another 30 seconds, until some tingling and distension are felt, ideally radiating to the entire abdomen.

Effect: Treat infertility, amenorrhea, menstrual disorder, dysmenorrhea, uterus prolapse, appendicitis and pelvic inflammation and orchitis.

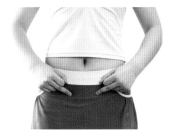

Press and knead the Guilai point.

7. Pressing and Kneading the Shuidao Point

Location: Three cun below the navel and two cun from the frontal middle line.

Method: Sit upright or lie on the back. First use two thumbs to press and knead the Shuidao point of the same side for 30 seconds. Then continue for another two minutes, until some tingling and distension are felt, ideally radiating to the entire abdomen.

Effect: Treat distension in the lower abdomen, difficult urination, hernia, dysmenorrhea and infertility.

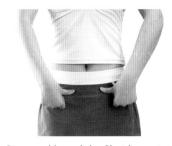

Press and knead the Shuidao point.

8. Pressing and Kneading the Baichongwo Point

Location: One cun above the Xuehai point.

Method: Sit upright. Use two thumbs to forcefully press and knead the Baichongwo point of both sides for two minutes, until some tingling and distension are felt as the best effect.

Effect: Treat intestinal ascariasis, scabies, hives, eczema, neurodermatitis, skin itch and scabies as well as problems with the knee joints and surrounding soft tissues.

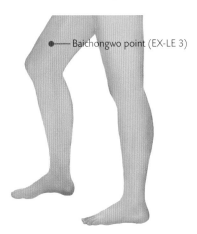

Baichongwo point (EX-LE 3)

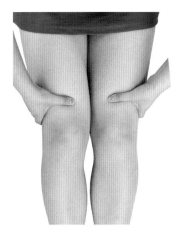

Press and knead the Baichongwo point.

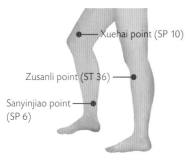

Location of the Xuehai, Zusanli and Sanyinjiao points.

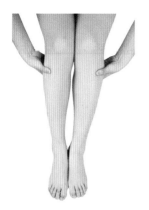

Press and knead the Zusanli point.

9. Pressing and Kneading the Sanyinjiao Point

Location: At the rear edge of the shinbone, three cun above the ankle.

Method: Sit upright and place one shin on the opposite thigh. Use the thumb to press, rub and knead the Sanyinjiao point for about two minutes until tingling and distension are felt in the part concerned as the best effect.

Effect: Cure insomnia, palpitation, high blood pressure, menstrual disorder, dysmenorrhea, impotence and nocturnal emission.

10. Pressing and Kneading the Zusanli Point

Location: About three cun below the knee on the outer side of the tibia.

Method: Sit upright. Use both thumbs to press the point on both sides, with the four fingers alongside the outer side of the lower leg, pressing and kneading outward 20 to 40 times, until some tingling and distension are felt as the best effect.

Effect: Treat diarrhea, abdominal pain and distension, lack of appetite, constipation, hiccups, vomiting, anemia, low blood pressure, menopause syndrome and waist-leg pain.

11. Pressing and Kneading the Xuehai Point

Location: The Xuehai point is in a cavity about two cun away from the inner upper corner of the patella, when the knee is bent. For Liangqiu point, it is in a cavity two cun above the outer upper corner of the patella.

Method: Sit upright. Use the pads of the thumbs to forcefully press and knead the Xuehai point of the same side for two minutes, until some tingling and distension are felt as the best effect.

Effect: Cure low blood pressure, inadequate vital energy and blood, anemia, dizziness and visual dizziness, menstrual disorder, dysmenorrhea, amenorrhea, hives, eczema, rough skin, skin itch and knee-joint pain.

Tips
- In order to get rid of the itching, some people scratch or wash the vulva with salty water or hot water, which cannot cure it, but instead makes it worse.
- Pay attention to hygiene during menstruation and wash the vulva with warm water every evening.
- Cleanse the vulva each time after urinating.

56 | Hyperplasia of the Mammary Glands

This is a common disease among women, referring to the hyperplasia of the epithelium of the mammary glands and the fiber tissues, degenerative pathological changes in the structure of the catheter and the lobules of the mammary glands, as well as the growth of progressive connective tissues.

It is associated with endocrine imbalance, in addition to relating closely to mental factors, ways of life and environmental factors. These may include bearing children after the age of 30, the absence of breast-feeding, martial disharmony, consuming products with hormones, or wearing a very tight bra that compresses lymph and blood circulation. After the onset of hyperplasia of the mammary glands, there may be tumors of the mammary glands with malicious pathological changes if not enough attention is paid.

Symptoms

These are divided into three types: breast pain, adenosis and cystic hyperplasia of the mammary glands.

Breast pain: Periodic breast pain is mostly related to the cycle of menstruation. It is obvious before menstruation and becomes alleviated after menstruation. No lumps can be felt in the mammary glands. In most cases it is a widely spread granular area of thickened tissues, hence also being called granular mammary glands.

Adenosis of the mammary glands: It is often marked by a painful local lump in one side of the mammary glands, and sometimes in both sides. The pain is associated with the cycle of menstruation. It most occurs in the outer upper part of the breasts, with a quite small lump of one to three centimeters in diameter. As it is not hard, it is not clearly separated from its surrounding tissues.

Cystic hyperplasia of the mammary glands: A breast lump, it is mostly seen among middle-aged women. It can be a fairly big single lump shaped like a round ball with a smooth surface, being cystic or substantial. Or it may feature a number of cystic tubers. About one-third of patients suffer from pain, at least when touched, in the early stage, but which is mostly not obvious. Sometimes there will be liquid coming from the nipples.

Target Acupoints

Shoulder, back and waist: Ganshu (BL 18).
Chest and abdomen: Danzhong (RN 17), Wuyi (ST 15), Rugen (ST 18), Yingchuang (ST 16), Qimen (LV 14), Riyue (GB 24).
Legs: Zusanli (ST 36), Sanyinjiao (SP 6), Taichong (LV 3).

Recommended Massage

1. Pressing the Ganshu Point

Location: 1.5 cun away from the ninth thoracic spinal process on the inner side of the scapula.

Method: Sit upright. Use the knuckles of the four fingers to knead the Ganshu point for about two minutes until tingling and distension are felt.

Effect: Treat distension and pain of both sides of the chest, breast pain with swelling, waist-back pain, agitation, irritability, indigestion and aversion to food, neurasthenia, hepatitis, jaundice (icterus), nausea, vomiting, lack of appetite and dizziness.

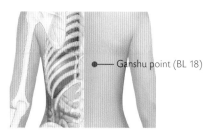
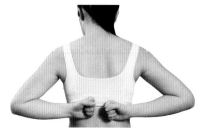

Ganshu point (BL 18)

Press the Ganshu point.

2. Pressing and Kneading the Wuyi Point

Location: In the second intercostal space directly above the nipple.

Method: Sit upright or lie on the back. Use the pad of the index finger to press and knead the Wuyi point for two minutes, until some tingling and distension are felt as the best effect.

Effect: Cure chest distension and pain, breast inflammation, breast distension and pain, hyperplasia of the mammary glands, asthma and cough, including that with pus and blood.

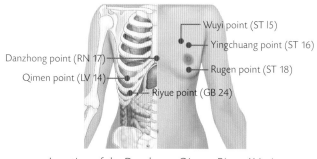

Wuyi point (ST 15)
Yingchuang point (ST 16)
Danzhong point (RN 17)
Rugen point (ST 18)
Qimen point (LV 14)
Riyue point (GB 24)

Location of the Danzhong, Qimen, Riyue, Wuyi, Yingchuang and Rugen points.

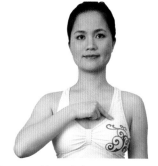

Press and knead the Wuyi point.

3. Palm Kneading the Danzhong Point

Location: Directly in the middle of the chest between the nipples.

Method: Use the thenar eminence of the left hand or the palm heel against the Danzhong point, kneading it 30 to 40 times. Then use the right hand to knead 30 to 40 times, until distension and numbness radiate to the chest as the best effect.

Effect: Cure difficulty in breathing, cough, chest pain, hyperplasia of the mammary glands, breast pain, lactation problems, palpitation and obesity.

4. Pressing and Kneading the Rugen Point

Location: In the fifth intercostal space at the base of the breast, directly under the nipple.

Method: Lie on the back. Use the thumb pad to press and knead the point, with the rest of the fingers helping to fix it. Keep the thumb kneading back and forth for two to three minutes until obvious tingling and distension are felt, along with comfort in the chest and breasts.

Effect: Cure chest pain, chest distress, breast distension and pain, agalactia, asthma and continuous hiccups.

5. Pressing and Kneading the Yingchuang Point

Location: In the third intercostal space above the breast central line.

Method: Sit upright or lie on the back. Use the thumb to press and knead the point for two minutes. Then do it for another two minutes with moderate force, until some tingling and distension are felt as the best effect.

Effect: Clear the chest and promote lactation, stop cough and eliminate swelling, as well as cure chest pain, with a particularly good effect on curing breast distension, including after giving birth or fever.

6. Pressing and Kneading the Qimen Point

Location: In the sixth intercostal space directly below the nipple.

Method: Sit upright or lie on the back. Use the pad of the middle finger to press and knead the Qimen point for two minutes with moderate force, until some tingling, distension and slight warmth are felt as the best effect.

Effect: Cure menstrual disorder, endometritis, abdominal pain, diarrhea, nausea, vomiting, liver pain, cholecystalgia and fatty liver disease.

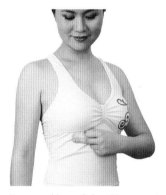

Press and knead the Qimen point.

7. Pressing and Kneading the Riyue Point

Location: In the seventh intercostal space directly below the nipple.

Method: Sit upright or lie on the back. Use the pad of the thumb to press and knead the Riyue point for two minutes, with the four fingers placed on ribs with moderate force, until some tingling, distension and slight warmth are felt as the best effect.

Effect: Treat cholecystitis, gallstones, biliary ascarids, hepatitis, gastric and duodenal ulcer, intercostal nerve pain, phrenospasm and shingles.

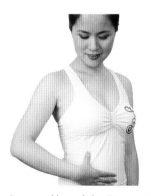

Press and knead the Riyue point.

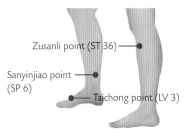

Zusanli point (ST 36)

Sanyinjiao point (SP 6)

Taichong point (LV 3)

Location of the Zusanli, Sanyinjiao and Taichong points.

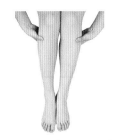

Press and knead the Zusanli point.

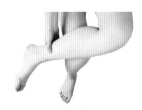

Press and knead the Sanyinjiao point.

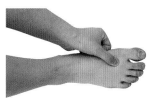

Press and knead the Taichong point.

8. Pressing and Kneading the Zusanli Point

Location: About three cun below the knee on the outer side of the tibia.

Method: Sit upright. Use the tips of two thumbs to press the Zusanli point on both sides respectively for one minute with gradually increasing force.

Effect: Promote the digestion and absorption of the stomach and intestines, enhance glycogen metabolism and improve physique.

9. Pressing and Kneading the Sanyinjiao Point

Location: At the rear edge of the shinbone, three cun above the ankle.

Method: Sit upright and place one shin on the opposite thigh. Use the thumb to press, rub and knead the Sanyinjiao point for about two minutes until tingling and distension are felt in the part concerned as the best effect.

Effect: Cure insomnia, palpitation, high blood pressure, menstrual disorder, dysmenorrhea, impotence and nocturnal emission.

10. Pressing and Kneading the Taichong Point

Location: On the foot in a notch between the first and second metatarsal bones.

Method: Sit upright. Use the thumb tip to press, rub and knead the Taichong point for about two minutes and then press for another 30 seconds until tingling and distension are felt in the part concerned as the best effect.

Effect: Cure headache with distension, dizziness, migraine, menstrual disorder including dysmenorrhea and amenorrhea, and breast pain with distension.

Tips

In order to check for diseases of the mammary glands, women over the age of 25 should self-examine their breasts each month:
- Stand in front of the mirror after bathing with arms akimbo, and observe whether the skin of both breasts is abnormal or if there is a depressed nipple.
- Then use the finger pad to move slowly over the breast clockwise or counterclockwise. Do not press or pinch it, to prevent normal tissues from being mistaken for lumps.

57 | Female Infertility

There are two kinds. Primary infertility is when a woman fails to become pregnant after two years of normal sexual activity without contraception. Secondary infertility is when a woman fails to become pregnant for two years after abortion or giving birth, again while having normal sexual activity without contraception.

Infertility is caused by the failure of endocrine function within the ovary or abnormal oogenesis (development of the fertilized egg), as well as an abnormal vaginal tract, resulting in impediment to the merger of sperm and egg or impediment to the implantation of the embryo.

Symptoms

As described above it is the failure to become pregnant despite sexual activity without adopting contraceptive for two years, given that the male partner has normal reproductive functions.

Target Acupoints

Shoulder, back and waist: Ganshu (BL 18), Pishu (BL 20), Shenshu (BL 23).
Chest and abdomen: Qihai (RN 6), Guanyuan (RN 4), Zhongji (RN 3), Zigong (EX-CA 1), Qugu (RN 2), Guilai (ST 29), Huangshu (KI 16).
Legs: Sanyinjiao (SP 6), Xuehai (SP 10), Fenglong (ST 40), Taichong (LV 3), Fuliu (KI 7), Ligou (LV 5).

Recommended Massage

1. Pressing the Ganshu Point
Location: 1.5 cun away from the ninth thoracic spinal process on the inner side of the scapula.

Method: Sit upright. Use the knuckles of the four fingers to knead the Ganshu point for about two minutes until tingling and distension are felt.

Effect: Treat distension and pain of both sides of the chest, breast pain with swelling, waist-back pain, agitation, irritability, indigestion and aversion to food, neurasthenia, hepatitis, jaundice (icterus), nausea, vomiting, lack of appetite and dizziness.

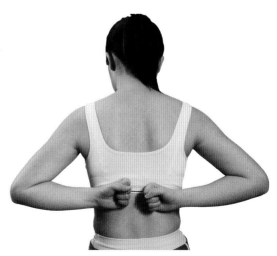

Press the Ganshu point.

2. Pressing and Kneading the Pishu Point

Location: At the point 1.5 cun away horizontally from the eleventh thoracic vertebra.

Method: Sit or stand. Use both middle fingers to press the Pishu point, with the thumb against the ribs, forcefully pressing and kneading for two minutes. Or with a clenched fist, use the index knuckle to press and knead the Pishu point for two minutes. Alternatively you may use a hollow fist to knead and rub it for two minutes, until some tingling and distension are felt.

Effect: Cure nausea, vomiting, abdominal distension, diarrhea, hemafecia (bloody stool) and jaundice.

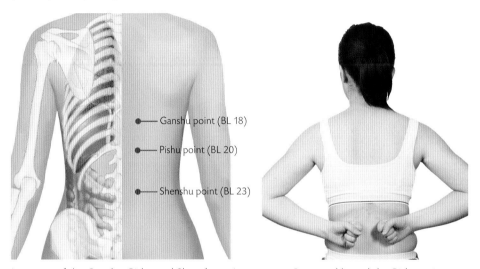

Location of the Ganshu, Pishu and Shenshu points.   Press and knead the Pishu point.

3. Pressing and Kneading the Shenshu Point

Location: 1.5 cun horizontally from the second lumbar spinal process.

Method: Lie on the back or sit upright. Use the two middle fingers to forcefully press and knead the Shenshu point of both sides 30 to 50 times, keeping the thumbs by the ribs. Or, with a clenched fist, use the knuckle of the index finger to press and knead the Shenshu point 30 to 50 times. You might also try using a loose fist to knead and rub 30 to 50 times, until some warmth is felt as the best effect.

Effect: Treat waist tingling and leg pain, lumbar muscle strain, lumbar disc herniation, leg swelling, fatigue all over the body, impotence, nocturnal emission, premature ejaculation and menstrual disorder.

4. Pressing and Kneading the Guanyuan Point

Location: About three cun below the navel.

Method: Sit upright or lie on the back. First use the index or middle finger to press the point for 30 seconds. Then continue to press and knead it for another two minutes, until some tingling and distension are felt as the best effect.

Effect: Cure abdominal pain and distension, menstrual disorder, dysmenorrhea, amenorrhea, nocturnal emission and impotence.

5. Pressing and Kneading the Qihai Point

Location: About 1.5 cun below the navel.

Method: Use the tips of the index and middle finger to press and knead the point for two minutes, until warmth is felt as the best effect.

Effect: Cure abdominal pain and distension, constipation or diarrhea, menstrual disorder, dysmenorrhea, amenorrhea.

6. Pressing and Kneading the Zhongji Point

Location: Four cun below the navel.

Method: Stand or lie on the back. First use the middle or index finger to press and knead the point for two minutes. Then continue to press it for another 30 seconds, until some tingling and distension are felt as the best effect.

Effect: Cure difficulty in urinating, leukorrhagia, amenorrhea, menstrual disorder, cold feeling and pain before menstruation, facial edema and lower-limb edema.

7. Pressing and Kneading the Zigong Point

Location: Four cun below the navel and three cun away from the frontal middle line.

Method: Stand or lie on the back. Use the thumbs to press the Zigong point of the same side for 30 seconds. Then continue to press and knead for another two minutes, until some tingling and distension are felt, ideally radiating to the entire abdomen.

Effect: Treat dysmenorrhea, menstrual disorder, profuse uterine bleeding, infertility and uterus prolapse.

8. Palm Kneading the Qugu Point

Location: Right on the frontal line, down from the navel at the upper line of the pubic bone.

Method: Stand or lie on the back. Use the right palm heel to press and knead the Qugu point for two minutes, with the left palm heel placed on the back of the right hand, until some tingling and distension are felt.

Effect: Cure menstrual disorder, uterine prolapse, urethritis, urinary retention, endometritis, cervix erosion, chronic pelvic inflammation, uterine inertia, dysmenorrhea, amenorrhea and leukorrhagia.

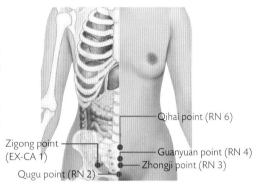

Zigong point (EX-CA 1)
Qihai point (RN 6)
Guanyuan point (RN 4)
Zhongji point (RN 3)
Qugu point (RN 2)

Location of the Zigong, Qihai, Guanyuan, Zhongji and Qugu points.

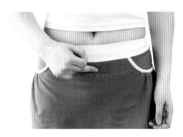

Press and knead the Zhongji point.

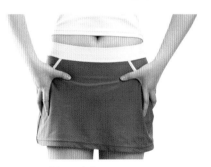

Press and knead the Zigong point.

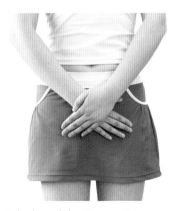

Palm knead the Qugu point.

9. Pressing and Kneading the Guilai Point

Location: Four cun below the navel and two cun away from the frontal middle line.

Method: Sit upright or lie on the back. Use two middle fingers to press and knead the Guilai points of both sides for two minutes. Then continue to press for another 30 seconds, until some tingling and distension are felt, ideally radiating to the entire abdomen.

Effect: Treat infertility, amenorrhea, menstrual disorder, dysmenorrhea, uterus prolapse, appendicitis and pelvic inflammation.

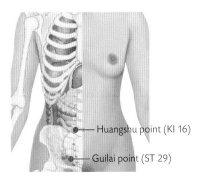

Huangshu point (KI 16)

Guilai point (ST 29)

Location of the Huangshu and Guilai points.

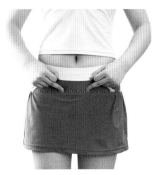

Press and knead the Guilai point.

10. Pressing and Kneading the Huangshu Point

Location: At the point 0.5 cun on either side of the navel.

Method: Use the middle or index finger to press and knead the point for about two minutes, until some tingling and distension are felt.

Effect: Cure physiological discomfort, waist pain and cold feeling.

11. Pressing and Kneading the Sanyinjiao Point

Location: At the rear edge of the shinbone, three cun above the ankle.

Method: Sit upright and place one shin on the opposite thigh. Use the thumb to press, rub and knead the Sanyinjiao point for about two minutes until tingling and

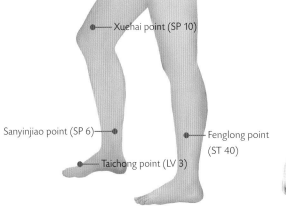

Xuehai point (SP 10)

Sanyinjiao point (SP 6)

Fenglong point (ST 40)

Taichong point (LV 3)

Location of the Xuehai, Sanyinjiao, Tiachong and Fenglong points.

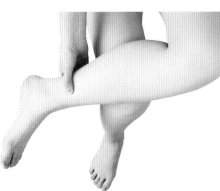

Press and knead the Sanyinjiao point.

distension are felt in the part concerned as the best effect.

Effect: Cure insomnia, palpitation, high blood pressure, menstrual disorder, dysmenorrhea.

12. Pressing and Kneading the Xuehai Point

Location: In a cavity about two cun away from the inner upper corner of the patella, when the knee is bent.

Method: Sit upright. Use the pads of the thumbs to forcefully press and knead the Xuehai point of the same side for two minutes, until some tingling and distension are felt as the best effect.

Effect: Cure low blood pressure, inadequate vital energy and blood, anemia, dizziness and visual dizziness, menstrual disorder, dysmenorrhea, amenorrhea, hives, eczema, rough skin, skin itch and knee-joint pain.

13. Pressing and Kneading the Fenglong Point

Location: Eight cun above the ankle tip.

Method: Sit upright. Use the thumb pad to press and knead the Fenglong points on both sides for two minutes, until tingling and distension are felt as the best effect.

Effect: Chiefly serve to treat mental disorders such as hysteria, insomnia and headache, as well as diseases of the circulatory system, such as high blood pressure, cerebral hemorrhage and the aftereffect of cerebrovascular diseases. It is beneficial for diseases of the respiratory system, such as acute and chronic bronchitis, asthma and pleurisy, as well as diseases of the digestive system, such as hepatitis, appendicitis, and constipation. In addition it can cure urine retention, addiction to smoking, obesity, leg-knee tingling and pain, and shoulder periarthritis.

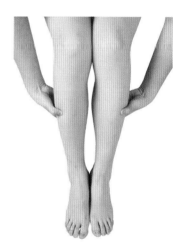

Press and knead the Fenglong point.

14. Pressing and Kneading the Taichong Point

Location: On the foot in a notch between the first and second metatarsal bones.

Method: Sit upright. Use the thumb tip to press, rub and knead the Taichong point for about two minutes and then press for another 30 seconds until tingling and distension are felt in the part concerned as the best effect.

Effect: Cure headache with distension, dizziness, migraine, menstrual disorder including dysmenorrhea and amenorrhea, and breast pain with distension.

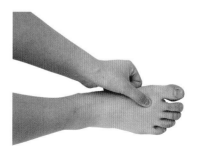

Press and knead the Taichong point.

15. Pressing and Kneading the Fuliu Point

Location: Two cun above the inner ankle tip right above the Taixi point.

Method: Use the pads of the index, middle and ring fingers of both hands to press and knead the point until warmth is felt in the part concerned. Or use two hands to rub the point back and forth; or massage in a circular motion.

Effect: Nourish the kidneys and yin energy, and clear channels within the body, as well as treat nephritis, neurasthenia, decline of energy and memory, cold hands and feet, and hand-foot edema.

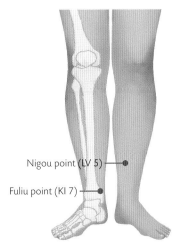

Nigou point (LV 5)

Fuliu point (KI 7)

Location of the Nigou and Fuliu points.

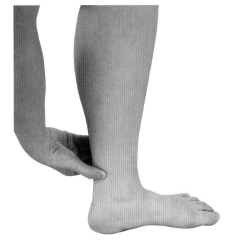

Press and knead the Fuliu point.

16. Pressing and Kneading the Nigou Point

Location: Five cun above the tip of the medial malleolus in the inner side of the calf.

Method: Use the thumb pad to press and knead the point with a little heavier force downward. Then slowly knead it in a moderate circular way, while the other fingers are placed beside the point to help the thumb exert force.

Effect: Treat tibia tingling and distension, menstrual disorder, genital itching, uterus prolapse, hernia, testicle distension and pain, endometritis and uterine prolapse.

Tips
- Infertility is one of the aftereffects of many gynecological diseases. A considerable number of cases of infertility can be prevented. Therefore timely treatment should be undertaken regarding gynecological diseases such as irregular menstruation.
- Try to avoid unwanted pregnancy and abortion, which may lead to secondary infertility or habitual abortion.

58 | Dark Circles

The skin around the eyes is very thin and full of blood vessels. This skin will become bluish-purple when blood does not circulate smoothly, leading to the lack of oxygen. Consequently there seems to be a dark circle.

Too much make-up, increased pressure and staying up late will lead to a dark circle. If it remains dark for a long time, it will be a morbid state that is often related to dysfunction of the endocrine system and metabolism, dysfunction of the adrenal cortex, pathological changes of vascular cardiology, blocked micro-circulation or chronic wasting diseases such as pathological diseases, requiring timely diagnosis and treatment.

Symptoms

The dark circles can be dark blue or dark brown.

Dark-blue circle: It often occurs among people over 20 years old, resulting from an abnormal daily schedule. It is caused by slow flow of blood within micro-blood vessels in the skin around the eyes, increase of oxygen consumption due to the increase of the amount of blood, and a large increase of blood that has been depleted of oxygen (anoxia). Therefore the skin looks dark blue.

Dark-brown circle: It is related to aging. Sun exposure over a long time leads to the precipitation of pigments around the eyes, gradually bringing about dark-brown circles that cannot be eliminated. In addition slow metabolism of dark pigments caused by static blood and excessive dry skin also results in the formation of dark-brown circles.

Target Acupoints

Head and neck: Jingming (BL 1), Tongziliao (GB 1), Sibai (ST 2), Yuyao (EX-HN 4), Sizhukong (SJ 23), Cuanzhu (BL 2), Chengqi (ST 1).
Arms: Hegu (LI 4).
Legs: Zusanli (ST 36).

Recommended Massage

1. Pressing and Kneading the Jingming Point
Location: In the depression over the inner corner of the eye.

Method: Lie on the back or sit upright. Use the thumb tip, index finger or middle finger to press the Jingming point of the affected side, pressing the inner upper part for two minutes until some tingling and distension are felt as the best effect.

Effect: Ease fatigue and restore eyesight, as well as treat bloodshot eyes, red swelling, edema, glaucoma and cataract. In addition it can ease nasal congestion when accompanied by massage of acupoints around the nose.

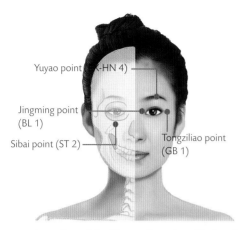

Location of the Yuyao, Jingming, Sibai and Tongziliao points.

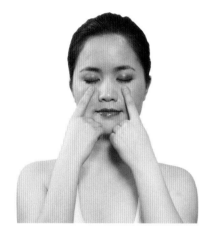

Press and knead the Sibai point.

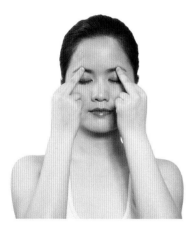

Press and knead the Yuyao point.

2. Pressing and Kneading the Tongziliao Point

Location: At the point 0.5 cun laterally outside of the outer canthus.

Method: Use the pad of the index finger to press the Tongziliao point of the affected side. When there is tingling and pain, increase force to press and knead for two minutes, radiating the tingling and distension to the eyes.

Effect: It has a very good effect on curing headache, dizziness, seeing stars, visual fatigue, eye itch and conjunctival congestion. It is also an important acupoint for eye beauty therapy.

3. Pressing and Kneading the Sibai Point

Location: Directly below the pupil, in a cavity below the orbit.

Method: Use the pads of the middle fingers to press the Sibai point on both sides. When there is tingling and pain, gradually increase force, pressing and kneading for about two minutes, so that the radiating tingling and distension reaches to the eyes.

Effect: It has a very good effect on symptoms caused by facioplegia such as failure to open and close the eyes, pain near the cheeks, trigeminal pain, myopia, visual fatigue and giddiness. In addition it is also an acupoint frequently used in facial beauty therapy.

4. Pressing and Kneading the Yuyao Point

Location: Directly above the pupil in the middle of each eyebrow.

Method: Use the pads of the two index or middle fingers to gently press and knead the Yuyao points above the eyes for two minutes, until tingling and distension are felt as the best effect.

Effect: Cure forehead pain, drooping eyelids, red and swollen eyes with pain, slight corneal opacity and myopia.

5. Pressing and Kneading the Sizhukong Point

Location: In a cavity near the outer eyebrow tip.

Method: Use the pad of the index finger to press the Sizhukong point. When there are tingling and distension, proceed from light to heavy force for about two minutes, ideally until the effect radiates to the eyes.

Effect: It is often used in eye beauty therapy, serving to prevent lines and dark circles, in addition to curing headache, swollen and painful eyes, twitching eyelids and toothache.

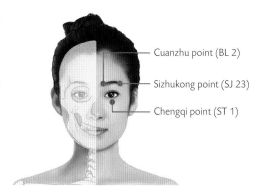

Cuanzhu point (BL 2)

Sizhukong point (SJ 23)

Chengqi point (ST 1)

Location of the Sizhukong, Cuanzhu and Chengqi points.

6. Pressing and Kneading the Cuanzhu Point

Location: In a cavity where the inner eyebrow starts.

Method: Use the pad of the index finger to press the Cuanzhu point of the affected side. When there are tingling and distension, proceed from light to heavy force for about two minutes until tingling and distension radiate to the eyes.

Effect: It has a very good effect on eye tearing, dizziness, visual fatigue, eye edema, conjunctivitis, cheek pain, headache and high blood pressure. The Cuanzhu point is also often used in facial beauty treatment.

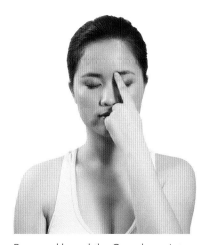

Press and knead the Cuanzhu point.

7. Pressing and Kneading the Chengqi Point

Location: Directly below the pupil, between the lower edge of the eyeball and the eye socket.

Method: Lie on the back or sit upright. Use the pad of the index finger to press and knead the margin in the middle of the suborbital part of the affected side. Continue for two minutes, until some tingling and distension are felt as the best effect.

Effect: Prevent tears caused by wind, myopia, nyctalopia, twitching eyelids, deviated mouth and eyes (facial paralysis) and facial convulsion.

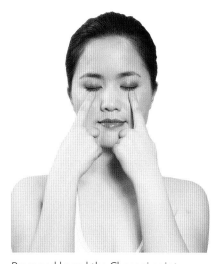

Press and knead the Chengqi point.

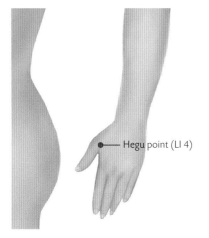

Location of the Hegu point.

8. Pinching and Kneading the Hegu Point
Location: In the highest point on the back of the hand between the thumb base and the base of the index finger (in the webbing between these two fingers).

Method: Use the thumb tip of one hand to pinch the Hegu point on the other hand for about one minute, and continue pinching and kneading for about two minutes, until some tingling and distension are felt as the best effect.

Effect: Treat cold, runny nose, headache, toothache, acne, visual fatigue, sore throat, tinnitus and hiccups.

9. Pressing the Zusanli Point
Location: About three cun below the knee on the outer side of the tibia.

Method: Use the tips of both thumbs to press the Zusanli points of both sides for one minute, proceeding from light to heavy force.

Effect: Promote gastric and intestinal digestion and absorption, enhance glycogen metabolism and reinforce physique.

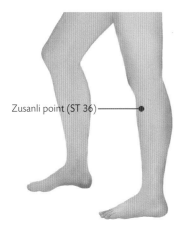
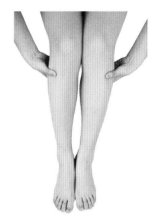

Press the Zusanli point.

Tips

Generally speaking an occasional dark circle is acceptable, as long as one adjusts the rhythm of daily life, avoids fatigue and gently massages the skin around eyes, making the color of the circle lighten or disappear.

59 | Eye Pouch

They are caused by fat reduction within the eye socket and imbalance of nutrition. They are also related to unavoidable aging.

Once formed, eye pouches, or eye bags, are not apt to disappear. They not only affect facial appearance but also blood circulation of the eyes, reducing the gel fiber property of the deep inner layer of the skin and gradually diminishing elasticity. This leads to loosened and wrinkled skin as well as fishtail lines radiating from the outer eye corners.

Symptoms

There are five kinds of eye pouches as follows:

Simple orbicularis muscle hypertrophy: Generally the skin is not loose. Eye pouches are close to the lower eyelid, spreading continuously in an arc form. Mostly caused by hereditary factors, they are often seen among young people.

Lower eyelid bulge of light and medium degrees: It is marked by excessive congenital development of orbital fat, which is often seen among young and middle-aged people.

Simple skin relaxation: There is no orbital relaxation but it is marked by skin relaxation of the lower eyelid and outer canthus without protruding orbital fat. There are some fine wrinkles around eyes. Simple skin relaxation is often seen among middle-aged people.

Lower eyelid bulge of a heavy degree coupled with skin relaxation: It is marked by relaxation of the skin, the orbicularis muscle and the orbit, leading to the fall of orbital fat. Those with serious cases suffer from ligament relaxation of the outer canthus, and separation of the eyelid from the eyeball often accompanied by tears. It is often seen among middle-aged and older people.

Skin relaxation coupled with a cavity between the lower-lid margin and infraorbital margin: In addition to skin relaxation, there appears a contraction of orbital fat and fat in front of the tarsus in the eyelid. It is often seen among middle-aged and older people.

Target Acupoints

Head and neck: Sibai (ST 2), Tongziliao (GB 1), Jingming (BL 1), Taiyang (EX-HN 5).
Legs: Yinlingquan (SP 9), Zusanli (ST 36), Sanyinjiao (SP 6).
Arms: Hegu (LI 4).

Recommended Massage

1. Pressing and Kneading the Sibai Point
Location: Directly below the pupil, in a cavity below the orbit.
Method: Use the pads of the index fingers to press the Sibai point on both sides. When there is tingling and pain, gradually increase force, pressing and kneading for

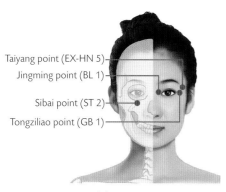

Taiyang point (EX-HN 5)
Jingming point (BL 1)
Sibai point (ST 2)
Tongziliao point (GB 1)

Location of the Taiyang, Jingming, Sibai and Tongziliao points.

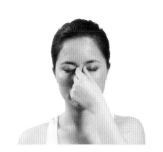

Press and knead the Jingming point.

about two minutes, so that the radiating tingling and distension reaches to the eyes.

Effect: It has a very good effect on symptoms caused by facioplegia such as failure to open and close the eyes, pain near the cheeks, trigeminal pain, myopia, visual fatigue and giddiness. In addition it is also an acupoint frequently used in facial beauty therapy.

2. Pressing and Kneading the Jingming Point

Location: In the depression over the inner corner of the eye.

Method: Lie on the back or sit upright. Use the thumb tip, index finger or middle finger to press the Jingming point of the affected side, pressing the inner upper part for two minutes until some tingling and distension are felt as the best effect.

Effect: Ease fatigue and restore eyesight, as well as treat bloodshot eyes, red swelling, edema, glaucoma and cataract. In addition it can ease nasal congestion when accompanied by massage of acupoints around the nose.

3. Pressing and Kneading the Tongziliao Point

Location: At the point 0.5 cun laterally outside of the outer canthus.

Method: Use the pad of the index finger to press the Tongziliao point of the affected side. When there is tingling and pain, increase force to press and knead for two minutes, radiating the tingling and distension to the eyes.

Effect: It has a very good effect on curing headache, dizziness, seeing stars, visual fatigue, eye itch and conjunctival congestion. It is also an important acupoint for eye beauty therapy.

4. Pressing and Kneading the Taiyang Point

Location: In the depression about one cun behind the space between the outer tip of the brow and outer eye corner.

Method: Sit upright or lie on the back. Use the pad of the index finger to press the Taiyang points on both sides of the head, rubbing and kneading for two minutes until you feel tingling and expansion in the acupoints. If rubbing and kneading of a larger area is required, or you need more force, use the thenar eminences.

Effect: Cure cold, headache, fever, dizziness, and red and swollen eyes with pain.

5. Pressing and Kneading the Yinlingquan Point

Location: In the depression on the inner edge of the shinbone below the knee.

Method: Sit upright. Use the thumb pads to press and knead the point for two minutes, with the four fingers grasping the rear of the leg, until tingling and distension are felt as the best effect.

Effect: Cure knee joint swelling and pain, abdominal distension, diarrhea, obesity, facial edema, edema all over the body, eyelid edema, eye pouches, difficult urination or urinary incontinence.

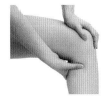

Press and knead the Yanglingquan point.

6. Pressing and Kneading the Zusanli Point
Location: About three cun below the knee on the outer side of the tibia.

Method: Sit upright. Use both thumbs to press the point on both sides, with the four fingers alongside the outer side of the lower leg, pressing and kneading outward 20 to 40 times, until some tingling and distension are felt as the best effect.

Effect: Treat diarrhea, abdominal pain and distension, lack of appetite, constipation, hiccups, vomiting, anemia, low blood pressure, menopause syndrome and waist-leg pain.

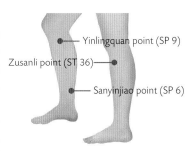

Location of the Yanglingquan, Zusanli and Sanyinjiao points.

7. Pressing and Kneading the Sanyinjiao Point
Location: At the rear edge of the shinbone, three cun above the ankle.

Method: Sit upright and place one shin on the opposite thigh. Use the thumb to press, rub and knead the Sanyinjiao point for about two minutes until tingling and distension are felt in the part concerned as the best effect.

Effect: Cure insomnia, palpitation, high blood pressure, menstrual disorder, dysmenorrhea, impotence and nocturnal emission.

8. Pinching and Kneading the Hegu Point
Location: In the highest point on the back of the hand between the thumb base and the base of the index finger (in the webbing between these two fingers).

Method: Sit upright or lie on the back. Use the thumb to press and knead the Hegu point while using the index finger to press its corresponding point on the palm 10 to 20 times alternately. Proceed from light to heavy force, until some tingling and distension are felt as the best effect.

Effect: Treat cold, runny nose, headache, toothache, acne, visual fatigue, sore throat, tinnitus and hiccups.

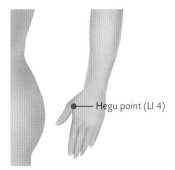

Location of the Hegu point.

Tips
In daily life the formation of eye pouches can be delayed if attention is paid to the care of eyes.

60 | Fishtail Lines

As time goes by, people after the age of 25 will experience aging skin and begin to have wrinkles, generally starting from the forehead, upper and lower eyelids, outer canthus, preauricular region, cheeks, neck, lower jaw and around the mouth. The contraction of the skin surface will form concave and convex stripes as the earliest sign of aging skin.

Fishtail lines refer to fine wrinkles appearing between the eye corners and temples. They are so named because their lines are similar to those of a fishtail. Acupoint massage can promote skin metabolism, discharge toxins inside the body, and prevent various aging diseases.

Symptoms

Fishtail lines often take place in middle-aged and older people, at varying lengths, depths, numbers and forms.

Target Acupoints

Head and face: Yangbai (GB 14), Touwei (ST 8), Yintang (EX-HN 3), Sizhukong (SJ 23), Tongziliao (GB 1), Taiyang (EX-HN 5), Shangxing (DU 23).
Arms: Hegu (LI 4).

Recommended Massage

1. Pressing and Kneading the Yangbai Point
Location: Directly in line with the pupil, one cun above the eyebrow on the forehead.

Method: Sit upright or lie on the back. Use two index fingers to gently press and knead the Yangbai points of both sides for about two minutes, until some tingling and distension are felt as the best effect.

Effect: An important acupoint for beautifying the forehead, it serves to cure forehead wrinkles, dark spots and drooping upper eyelids, with some curative effect on trifacial neuralgia, headache and visual fatigue.

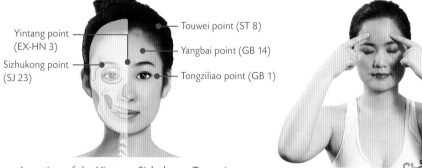

Yintang point (EX-HN 3)
Sizhukong point (SJ 23)
Touwei point (ST 8)
Yangbai point (GB 14)
Tongziliao point (GB 1)

Location of the Yintang, Sizhukong, Touwei, Yangbai and Tongziliao points.

Press and knead the Yangbai point.

2. Pushing and Massaging the Yintang Point

Location: At the central point right between the eyebrows.

Method: Sit upright or lie on the back. Use the pad of the middle finger to press and knead the Yintang point up and down for about two minutes.

Effect: Treat cold, insomnia, vascular headache, frontal sinusitis, supra-orbital neuralgia, acute and chronic rhinitis, nose bleeding, nasal polyp, acne rosacea, high blood pressure, neurasthenia, malaria, nervous vomiting, postpartum anemic fainting, eclampsia, febrile convulsion, facial convulsion, facioplegia, and acute and chronic conjunctivitis.

3. Pressing and Kneading the Touwei Point

Location: Front of the head at the hairline, 0.5 cun from the center line on both sides.

Method: Sit upright or lie on the back. Use the pad of the middle finger to rub and knead the Touwei point on both sides of the head. Continue for about two minutes and then press for 30 seconds, ideally until you feel the tingling and expansion radiate to the entire front of the head and both sides of the point.

Effect: Increase longevity, reduce wrinkles, and prevent hair from becoming sparse, split or gray, in addition to curing itchy scalp, migraine, forehead neuralgia, high blood pressure, conjunctivitis and decline of eyesight.

4. Pressing and Kneading the Sizhukong Point

Location: In a cavity near the outer eyebrow tip.

Method: Use the pad of the index finger to press the Sizhukong point. When there are tingling and distension, proceed from light to heavy force for about two minutes, ideally until the effect radiates to the eyes.

Effect: It is often used in eye beauty therapy, serving to prevent lines and dark circles, in addition to curing headache, swollen and painful eyes, twitching eyelids and toothache.

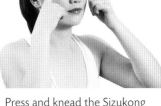

Press and knead the Sizukong point.

5. Pressing and Kneading the Tongziliao Point

Location: At the point 0.5 cun laterally outside of the outer canthus.

Method: Use the pad of the index finger to press the Tongziliao point of the affected side. When there is tingling and pain, increase force to press and knead for two minutes, radiating the tingling and distension to the eyes.

Effect: It has a very good effect on curing headache, dizziness, seeing stars, visual fatigue, eye itch and conjunctival congestion. It is also an important acupoint for eye beauty therapy.

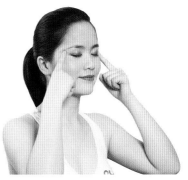

Press and knead the Tongziliao point.

6. Pressing and Kneading the Taiyang Point

Location: In the depression about one cun behind the space between the outer tip of the brow and outer eye corner.

Method: Sit upright or lie on the back. Use the pad of the index finger to press the Taiyang points on both sides of the head, rubbing and kneading for two minutes until you feel tingling and expansion in the acupoints. If rubbing and kneading of a larger area is required, or you need more force, use the thenar eminences.

Effect: Cure cold, headache, fever, dizziness, and red and swollen eyes with pain.

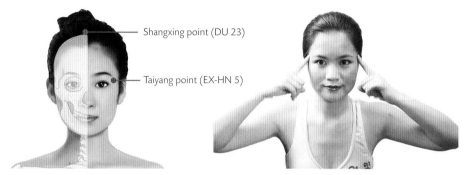

Shangxing point (DU 23)

Taiyang point (EX-HN 5)

Location of the Shangxing and Taiyang points.   Press and knead the Taiyang point.

7. Pressing and Kneading the Shangxing Point

Location: One cun above the frontal hairline on the median line of the head.

Method: Use the thumb or middle finger to press and knead the point clockwise for about two minutes, until some tingling and distension are felt in the forehead as the best effect.

Effect: Local massage serves to promote blood circulation and speed up metabolism. It can prevent hair from becoming dry, split and sparse while curing headache, head itch, fever, tears against wind, nose bleeding and nasosinusitis.

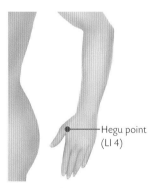

Hegu point (LI 4)

Location of Hegu point.

8. Pinching and Kneading the Hegu Point

Location: In the highest point on the back of the hand between the thumb base and the base of the index finger (in the webbing between these two fingers).

Method: Use the thumb tip of one hand to pinch the Hegu point on the other hand for about one minute, and continue pinching and kneading for about two minutes, until some tingling and distension are felt as the best effect.

Effect: Treat cold, runny nose, headache, toothache, acne, visual fatigue, sore throat, tinnitus and hiccups.

Tips

Regular care can delay the appearance of fishtail lines.

61 | Acne

It is one of the common diseases, often referred to as pimples. Eighty to ninety percent of people suffer from it at some point. It is mostly caused by undesirable life habits.

Symptoms

Mostly occurring on the face, it can also be seen on the upper part of the back, the chest, the rear of the neck and the buttocks among other places. People will feel slight itching or pain, lasting for a long time. Very often, it appears occasionally, with new ones forming constantly. Some cases may last for several years.

There are three kinds of acne:

Blackhead: It is follicular rash with a black dot at the center.

Whitehead: With a red color all around, white thick liquid can be squeezed out.

Small pimple: Neither a blackhead nor whitehead, it is small neutral color pimple.

In case of inflammation, acne can affect one's appearance. After disappearance there may be pigments or scars left behind, even severe scarring in serious cases.

In clinical practice, one or two cases with quite obvious symptoms are commonly seen, usually often accompanied by head-face seborrheic dermatitis. The face will look oily and shining, and there may be reddening of the skin in large areas covered with oily scabs.

Target Acupoints

Head and face: Quanliao (SI 18), Yingxiang (LI 20), Taiyang (EX-HN 5).
Shoulder, back and waist: Dazhui (RN 14), Ganshu (BL 18), Feishu (BL 13), Weishu (BL 21).
Arms: Quchi (LI 11), Hegu (LI 4).
Legs: Neiting (ST 44), Xuehai (SP 10).

Recommended Massage

1. Pressing and Kneading the Quanliao Point

Location: Directly in the lower part of the outer canthus, in a cavity of the lower margin of the cheekbone.

Method: Lie on the back or sit upright. Use the index or middle finger to press and knead the Quanliao point of the affected side for about 30 seconds. Then continue for two minutes, until some tingling and distension are felt in the part concerned and radiated to the entire face as the best effect.

Effect: Chiefly serve to treat toothache, trifacial neuralgia, mandibular arthritis, disLocation of lower jaw, convulsion of the zygomaxillary muscle, facial convulsion, facioplegia, tympanitis, dizziness and tinnitus.

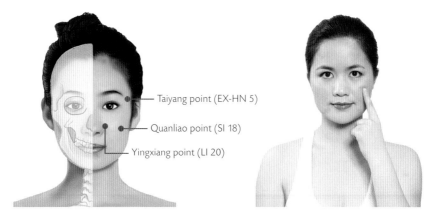

Location of the Taiyang, Quanliao and Yingxiang points.

Press and knead the Quanliao point.

2. Pressing and Kneading the Yingxiang Point

Location: Beside the wing of the nose, 0.5 cun away, in the nasolabial groove.

Method: Sitting upright, first use the index finger to press and knead the point for two minutes and then press for another 30 seconds, until some tingling and distension are felt as the best effect.

Effect: Excellent for easing various symptoms involving the nose, such as runny nose, nasal congestion, nose bleeding, nasosinusitis, decline of sense of smell, and chronic rhinitis. In addition this acupoint is also frequently used in cases of trifacial neuralgia and to treat the aftereffect of facial paralysis, as well as for facial beauty.

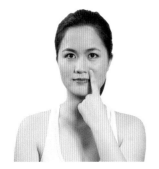

Press and knead the Yingxiang point.

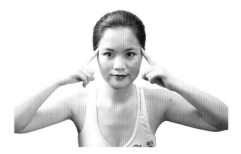

Press and knead the Taiyang point.

3. Pressing and Kneading the Taiyang Point

Location: In the depression about one cun behind the space between the outer tip of the brow and outer eye corner.

Method: Sit upright or lie on the back. Use the pad of the index finger to press the Taiyang points on both sides of the head, rubbing and kneading for two minutes until you feel tingling and expansion in the acupoints. If rubbing and kneading of a larger area is required, or you need more force, use the thenar eminences.

Effect: Cure cold, headache, fever, dizziness, and red and swollen eyes with pain.

4. Pressing the Dazhui Point

Location: Under the spinous process of the seventh cervical vertebrae.

Method: Sit upright. Use the tip of the middle finger to press the Dazhui point 20 or 30 times.

Effect: An important acupoint for health care, it serves to enhance the ability of preventing diseases, and to treat headache and neck pain, neck-shoulder syndrome, cervical spondylosis, fever, cold, asthma, malaria, chronic bronchitis, tuberculosis (TB) and epilepsy as well as cold limbs, shoulder-back cold pain and physical weakness caused by the lack of vital energy.

5. Pressing and Kneading the Ganshu Point

Location: 1.5 cun away from the ninth thoracic spinal process on the inner side of the scapula.

Method: Sit upright. Use the knuckles of the four fingers to knead the Ganshu point for about two minutes until tingling and distension are felt.

Effect: Treat distension and pain of both sides of the chest, breast pain with swelling, waist-back pain, agitation, irritability, indigestion and aversion to food, neurasthenia, hepatitis, jaundice (icterus), nausea, vomiting, lack of appetite and dizziness.

6. Pressing and Kneading the Feishu Point

Location: At the point 1.5 cun beside the third thoracic vertebra on the inner side of the scapula.

Method: Sit upright. First use the tip of the middle finger of the left hand to press and knead the Feishu point of the right side for two minutes. Then use the tip of the middle finger of the right hand to press and knead the Feishu point of the left side, ideally until warmth is felt.

Effect: Treat cold, cough, bronchitis, asthma, spontaneous perspiration, night sweating and back tingling and pain.

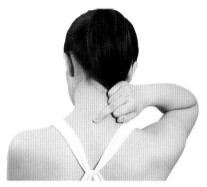

Press the Dazhui point.

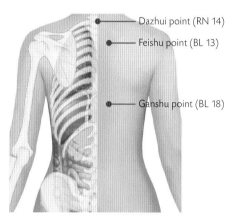

Dazhui point (RN 14)

Feishu point (BL 13)

Ganshu point (BL 18)

Location of the Dazhui, Feishu and Ganshu points.

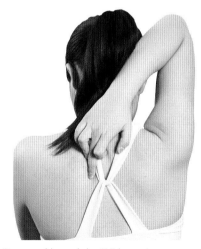

Press and knead the Feishu point.

7. Pressing and Kneading the Weishu Point

Location: About 1.5 cun below the spinous process of the twelfth thoracic vertebra.

Method: Sit upright. Use the middle finger knuckle to press and knead the point for two minutes, until some tingling and distension are felt as the best effect.

Effect: Treat all kinds of diseases and symptoms of the digestive system, such as acute gastritis, chronic gastritis, gastroptosis, stomach atony, abdominal distension, abdominal pain, lack of appetite, nausea and vomiting.

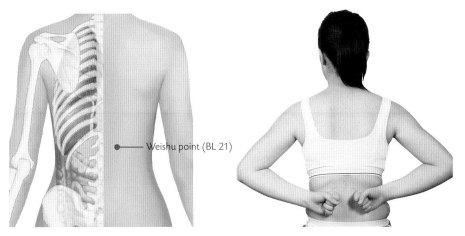

Weishu point (BL 21)

Press and knead the Weishu point.

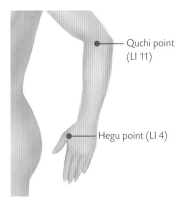

Quchi point
(LI 11)

Hegu point (LI 4)

Location of the Quchi and Hegu points.

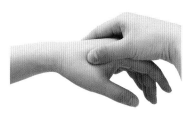

Pinch and knead the Hegu point.

8. Pinching and Pressing the Quchi Point

Location: With the elbow bent halfway, on the outer side of the cubital transverse crease.

Method: Sit upright with the arm bent halfway. Use the thumb of the other hand to pinch and press the Quchi point for one minute. Then press and knead for another two minutes, until some tingling and distension are felt.

Effect: Treat toothache, sore throat, migraine, dizziness, red face and eyes, acne, chloasma, hives, erysipelas and arm pain.

9. Pinching and Kneading the Hegu Point

Location: In the highest point on the back of the hand between the thumb base and the base of the index finger (in the webbing between these two fingers).

Method: Use the thumb tip of one hand to pinch the Hegu point on the other hand for about one minute, and continue pinching and kneading for about two minutes, until some tingling and distension are felt as the best effect.

Effect: Treat cold, runny nose, headache, toothache, acne, visual fatigue, sore throat, tinnitus and hiccups.

10. Pressing and Kneading the Neiting Point

Location: On the dorso-ventral boundary of the foot, in the rear of the toe web between the second and third toe.

Method: Sit upright. Use the index finger to press and knead the point, until some tingling and distension are felt as the best effect.

Effect: Reduce inner heat and tranquilize the spirit, in addition to curing toothache, sore throat, nose bleeding, bad breath, acid regurgitation, diarrhea, acne rosacea, swelling and pain of the back of the foot, and toe joint pain.

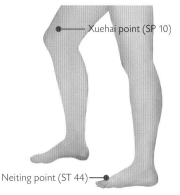

Xuehai point (SP 10)

Neiting point (ST 44)

Location of the Xuehai and Neiting points.

11. Pressing and Kneading the Xuehai Point

Location: In a cavity about two cun away from the inner upper corner of the patella, when the knee is bent.

Method: Sit upright. Use the pads of the thumbs to forcefully press and knead the Xuehai point of the same side for two minutes, until some tingling and distension are felt as the best effect.

Effect: Cure low blood pressure, inadequate vital energy and blood, anemia, dizziness and visual dizziness, menstrual disorder, dysmenorrhea, amenorrhea, hives, eczema, rough skin, skin itch and knee-joint pain.

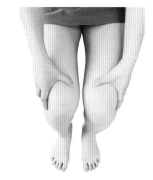

Press and knead the Xuehai point.

Tips

- It is better not to squeeze pimples, because there may be viruses on the fingers that will result in infection. Serious infection will lead to malignant boils, sores and bumpy patches. Scars of different sizes may be left behind after the affected skin is cured.
- After disinfection, well-trained doctors and nurses can completely get rid of some blackheads and purulent pimples.

62 | Rough and Dull Skin

It is caused by dead skin left behind on the face, skin allergy, use of improper cosmetics and staying up late. These factors can prevent the skin from completing normal metabolism, leading to rough and dull skin.

Symptoms
Coarse skin is often seen on the face or the back of the hand, accompanied by itching and flaking. The symptom is particularly obvious in dry seasons.

Target Acupoints
Head and neck: Yintang (EX-HN 3), Taiyang (EX-HN 5), Quanliao (SI 18).
Shoulder, back and waist: Feishu (BL 13), Weishu (BL 21), Ganshu (BL 18), Pishu (BL 20).
Legs: Xuehai (SP 10), Zusanli (ST 36), Sanyinjiao (SP 6).
Arms: Quchi (LI 11).

Recommended Massage
1. Pushing and Massaging the Yintang Point
Location: At the central point right between the eyebrows.

Method: Sit upright or lie on the back. Use the thumb to push the point, with the four fingers against the exterior of the eyes. Use the pad of the thumb to push to the hairline, repeating 20 to 30 times.

Effect: Cure headache, dizziness, visual fatigue, dark circles, forehead wrinkles, dull or dark color of the forehead, nasal congestion, acne rosacea and nasosinusitis.

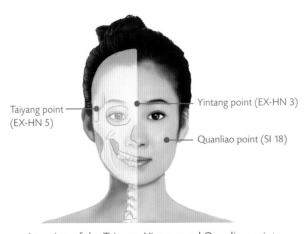

Taiyang point (EX-HN 5)

Yintang point (EX-HN 3)

Quanliao point (SI 18)

Location of the Taiyang, Yintang and Quanliao points.

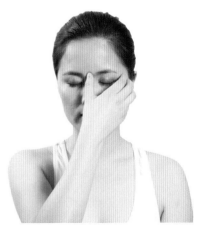

Push and massage the Yintang point.

2. Pressing and Kneading the Taiyang Point

Location: In the depression about one cun behind the space between the outer tip of the brow and outer eye corner.

Method: Sit upright or lie on the back. Use the pad of the index finger to press the Taiyang points on both sides of the head, rubbing and kneading for two minutes until you feel tingling and expansion in the acupoints. If rubbing and kneading of a larger area is required, or you need more force, use the thenar eminences.

Effect: Cure cold, headache, fever, dizziness, and red and swollen eyes with pain.

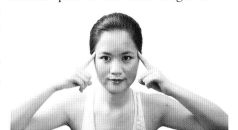

Press and knead the Taiyang point.

3. Pressing and Kneading the Quanliao Point

Location: Directly in the lower part of the outer canthus, in a cavity of the lower margin of the cheekbone.

Method: Lie on the back or sit upright. Use the index or middle finger to press and knead the Quanliao point of the affected side for about 30 seconds. Then continue for two minutes, until some tingling and distension are felt in the part concerned and radiated to the entire face as the best effect.

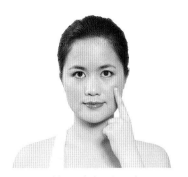

Press and knead the Quanliao point.

Effect: Chiefly serve to treat toothache, trifacial neuralgia, mandibular arthritis, disLocation of lower jaw, convulsion of the zygomaxillary muscle, facial convulsion, facioplegia, tympanitis, dizziness and tinnitus.

4. Pressing and Kneading the Feishu Point

Location: At the point 1.5 cun beside the third thoracic vertebra on the inner side of the scapula.

Method: Sit upright. First place the left palm heel on the Jianjing point on the right side, with the middle fingertip pressing, rubbing and kneading the Feishu point on the right side for two minutes. Then place the right palm heel on the Jianjing point on the left side, kneading until the part concerned feels hot as the best effect.

Effect: Treat cold, cough, bronchitis, asthma, spontaneous perspiration, night sweating and back tingling and pain.

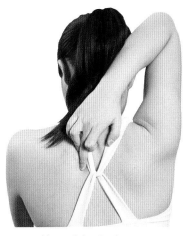

Press and knead the Feishu point.

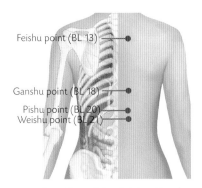

Feishu point (BL 13)

Ganshu point (BL 18)

Pishu point (BL 20)
Weishu point (BL 21)

Location of the Feishu, Ganshu, Pishu and Weishu points.

5. Pressing and Kneading the Weishu Point

Location: About 1.5 cun below the spinous process of the twelfth thoracic vertebra.

Method: Sit or stand. Use the middle fingers to press and knead the Weishu point of both sides (with the thumb against the ribs) forcefully for two minutes. Alternately make a fist and use the protruding index knuckle to press and knead it for two minutes. Or with a loose fist, press and rub the point for two minutes. In all cases some tingling and distension are felt as the best effect.

Effect: Treat all kinds of diseases and symptoms of the digestive system, such as acute gastritis, chronic gastritis, gastroptosis, stomach atony, abdominal distension, abdominal pain, lack of appetite, nausea and vomiting.

6. Pressing and Kneading the Ganshu Point

Location: 1.5 cun away from the ninth thoracic spinal process on the inner side of the scapula.

Method: Sit upright. Use the knuckles of the four fingers to knead the Ganshu point for about two minutes until tingling and distension are felt.

Effect: Treat distension and pain of both sides of the chest, breast pain with swelling, waist-back pain, agitation, irritability, indigestion and aversion to food, neurasthenia, hepatitis, jaundice (icterus), nausea, vomiting, lack of appetite and dizziness.

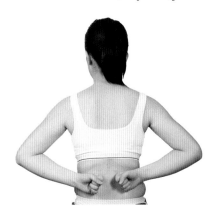

Press and knead the Pishu point.

7. Pressing and Kneading the Pishu Point

Location: At the point 1.5 cun away horizontally from the eleventh thoracic vertebra.

Method: Sit or stand. Use both middle fingers to press the Pishu point, with the thumb against the ribs, forcefully pressing and kneading for two minutes. Or with a clenched fist, use the index knuckle to press and knead the Pishu point for two minutes. Alternatively you may use a hollow fist to knead and rub it for two minutes, until some tingling and distension are felt.

Effect: Cure nausea, vomiting, abdominal distension, diarrhea, hemafecia (bloody stool) and jaundice.

8. Pressing and Kneading the Xuehai Point

Location: In a cavity about two cun away from the inner upper corner of the patella, when the knee is bent.

Method: Sit upright. Use the pads of the thumbs to forcefully press and knead the Xuehai point of the same side for two minutes, until some tingling and distension are felt as the best effect.

Effect: Cure low blood pressure, inadequate vital energy and blood, anemia, dizziness and visual dizziness, menstrual disorder, dysmenorrhea, amenorrhea, hives, eczema, rough skin, skin itch and knee-joint pain.

9. Pressing and Kneading the Sanyinjiao Point

Location: At the rear edge of the shinbone, three cun above the ankle.

Method: Sit upright and place one shin on the opposite thigh. Use the thumb to press, rub and knead the Sanyinjiao point for about two minutes until tingling and distension are felt in the part concerned as the best effect.

Effect: Cure insomnia, palpitation, high blood pressure, menstrual disorder, dysmenorrhea, impotence and nocturnal emission.

10. Pressing and Kneading the Zusanli Point

Location: About three cun below the knee on the outer side of the tibia.

Method: Sit upright. Use both thumbs to press the point on both sides, with the four fingers alongside the outer side of the lower leg, pressing and kneading outward 20 to 40 times, until some tingling and distension are felt as the best effect.

Effect: Cure pain around the knee joints, waist-leg pain, anemia, low blood pressure, diarrhea, abdominal pain, lack of appetite, constipation, vomiting, menopause syndrome and darkened skin without elasticity.

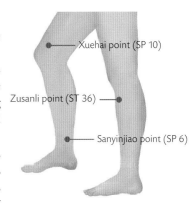

Location of the Xuehai, Sanyinjiao and Zusanli points.

11. Pinching and Kneading the Quchi Point

Location: With the elbow bent halfway, on the outer side of the cubital transverse crease.

Method: Sit upright with the arm bent halfway. Use the thumb of the other hand to pinch and press the Quchi point for one minute. Then press and knead for another two minutes, until some tingling and distension are felt.

Effect: Treat toothache, sore throat, migraine, dizziness, red face and eyes, acne, chloasma, hives, erysipelas and arm pain.

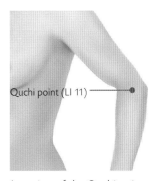

Location of the Quchi point.

> **Tips**
> - The early manifestation of some diseases, such as hepatitis, liver cirrhosis, nephritis and intestinal parasitic diseases, is marked by dull or discolored facial skin.
> - Malnutrition, and the lack of protein, vitamin C and vitamin A will also lead to dullness or discoloration.
> - Caffeine, pigments in beef and mutton, and tyrosine in bamboo shoots can be converted into dark pigments that lead to discoloration.

INDEX